Essential Physiology for Dental Students

Essential Physiology for Dental Students

Edited by

Kamran Ali
Associate Professor/Consultant in Oral Surgery
Peninsula Dental School University of Plymouth
UK

Elizabeth Prabhakar
Senior Lecturer in Medical Sciences, BARTS and the London School of
Medicine & Dentistry, Queen Mary University of London, Malta and a former
Lecturer in Physiology, Peninsula Schools of Medicine and Dentistry
University of Plymouth, UK

WILEY Blackwell

Registered Offices
John Wiley & Sons, Inc., 111 River Street, Hoboken, NJ 07030, USA
John Wiley & Sons Ltd, The Atrium, Southern Gate, Chi Chester, West Sussex, PO19 8SQ, UK

Editorial Office
9600 Garsington Road, Oxford, OX4 2DQ, UK

For details of our global editorial offices, customer services, and more information about Wiley products visit us at www.wiley.com.

Wiley also publishes its books in a variety of electronic formats and by print-on-demand. Some content that appears in standard print versions of this book may not be available in other formats.

Library of Congress Cataloging-in-Publication Data

Names: Ali, Kamran, editor. | Prabhakar, Elizabeth, editor.
Title: Essential physiology for dental students / edited by Kamran Ali, Elizabeth Prabhakar.
Description: Hoboken, NJ : John Wiley & Sons, 2019. | Includes bibliographical references and index. |
Identifiers: LCCN 2018022260 (print) | LCCN 2018023041 (ebook) | ISBN 9781119271611 (Adobe PDF) |
    ISBN 9781119271758 (ePub) | ISBN 9781119271710 (pbk.)
Subjects: | MESH: Physiological Phenomena
Classification: LCC RK76 (ebook) | LCC RK76 (print) | NLM QT 104 | DDC 617.60071/1–dc23
LC record available at https://lccn.loc.gov/2018022260

Cover Design: Wiley
Cover Image: © S.Y. Melina Kam

Set in 10/12pt AGaramondPro by SPi Global, Pondicherry, India
Printed and bound in Singapore by Markono Print Media Pte Ltd

10 9 8 7 6 5 4 3 2 1

To my mother and father, who are my role models
and taught me the core human values.

To my wife and children, for their extraordinary love
and support.

Kamran Ali

Dedicated to the memory of my late father,
who was an unending source of inspiration,
strength, and wisdom and for shaping my intellect.

To my mother and the rest of my family, for their
encouragement, love, and support.

Elizabeth Prabhakar

Contents

List of Contributors

Kamran Ali, Associate Professor/Consultant in Oral Surgery, Peninsula Dental School University of Plymouth, UK

Louise Belfield, Lecturer in Biomedical Sciences, Peninsula Dental School University of Plymouth, UK

Theresa Compton, Lecturer in Biomedical Sciences, Peninsula Dental School University of Plymouth, UK

Poorna Gunasekera, Associate Professor/Senior Lecturer in Biomedical Sciences, Peninsula Dental School University of Plymouth, UK

Elizabeth Prabhakar, Senior Lecturer in Medical Sciences, BARTS and the London School of Medicine & Dentistry, Queen Mary University of London, Malta and a former Lecturer in Physiology, Peninsula School of Medicine & Dentistry, University of Plymouth, UK

Mahwish Raja, General Dental Practitioner, Plymouth, UK

Vehid Salih, Associate Professor (Reader) in Oral and Dental Research, Peninsula Dental School University of Plymouth, UK

Feisal Subhan, Lecturer in Biomedical Sciences, Faculty of Medicine and Dentistry, University of Plymouth, UK

Preface

We are delighted to present a book on medical physiology written exclusively for a dental audience. It is envisaged that the book will be used not only in the early years of dental courses but also for preparation of postgraduate examinations in dentistry. Moreover, dentists and dental care professionals may also benefit from it to refresh and update their knowledge of physiology.

Physiology is a complex and challenging subject, and traditionally the dental students have learnt it from standard medical textbooks with limited reference to dentistry. A concerted effort has been made to provide the relevance of each topic area to dentistry so that dental students are able to relate the subject to their own clinical practice. We have not only focused on physiology but also tried to assimilate relevant concepts of allied subjects to achieve integration with other basic and clinical subjects.

A wide selection of online self-assessment questions accompany this text, and readers can use this resource not only to prepare for relevant examinations but also as a drive for their learning. While every effort has been made to discuss core topic areas in physiology comprehensively, it is suggested that readers explore additional resources to further enhance their understanding of the subject. Recommendations for additional online and text resources are listed at the end of each chapter.

Finally, we hope this book will be a useful addition to existing resources for dental students. We would like to express our utmost gratitude to all the contributors for sharing their knowledge and expertise in the subject.

Kamran Ali
PhD MMEd BDS (Hons) FDSRCS (Eng) FCPS (Pak)
FFDRCSI (Ire) FFDTEd FDSRCPS (Glasg) PFHEA

Elizabeth Prabhakar
PhD FHEA CBiol

About the Companion Website

Don't forget to visit the companion website for this book:

www.wiley.com/go/ali/physiology

There you will find valuable material designed to enhance your learning, including:
- MCQs
- EMQs
- Glossary
- List of abbreviations
- PowerPoint slides of figures

Scan this QR code to visit the companion website

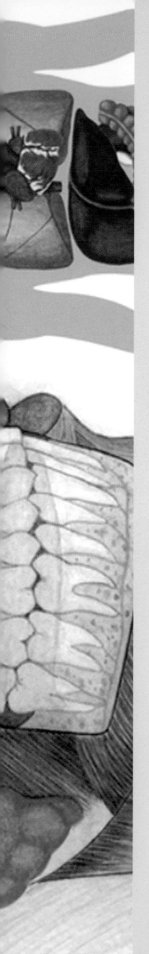

PART I

Introduction

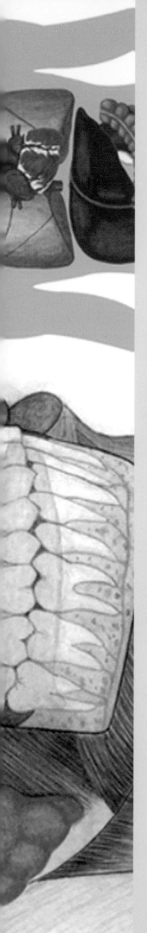

CHAPTER 1
The Cell: Structure and Function

Vehid Salih and Kamran Ali

Key Topics

- Overview of different types of living organisms
- Organisation of the human body
- Components of human cells
- Regeneration and repair

Learning Objectives

To demonstrate an understanding of the:

- Differences between prokaryotes and eukaryotes
- Structure and functions of the cell organelles
- Relevance of regeneration and repair to oral and dental tissues
- Potential applications of stem cells

Introduction

A cell is the fundamental structural, functional, and biological unit of all known living organisms (except viruses). Individual cells range from 1 to 100 μm and are visible only under a microscope as the human eye is unable to see anything smaller than 100 μm. Living organisms are described as unicellular (microorganisms) or multicellular (e.g. plants and animals). Unicellular organisms are also classified as *prokaryotes* and multicellular organisms as *eukaryotes*. Prokaryotes lack a nucleus and cytoplasmic organelles and are represented by bacteria. Eukaryotes have a nucleus as well as cytoplasmic organelles and include microorganisms such as fungi, protozoa, algae as well as animals and humans. Nevertheless, both types possess a cell membrane and contain deoxyribonucleic acid (DNA). Viruses are neither prokaryotes nor eukaryotes as they lack characteristics of living organisms,

Essential Physiology for Dental Students, First Edition. Edited by Kamran Ali and Elizabeth Prabhakar.
© 2019 John Wiley & Sons Ltd. Published 2019 by John Wiley & Sons Ltd.
Companion website: www.wiley.com/go/ali/physiology

apart from the ability to replicate. They are best regarded as obligate parasites as they can only replicate in living cells.

An adult human body comprises approximately 75–100 trillion cells, and more than 200 varieties of specialised cells have already been identified. The cells in the human body join to form tissues. Four basic human tissues include epithelium, connective tissue, nervous tissue, and muscle. Different tissues are grouped to form organs which in turn join to form various systems of the human body. The function of the human body is maintained by thousands of control systems at the level of cells, tissues, organs as well as systems allowing the body to maintain a constant internal environment, or *homeostasis*. Nevertheless, all physiological processes as well as disease mechanisms can be described at, and ascribed to, the cellular level. Cells are diverse and vary tremendously in their morphology and function. Figure 1.1 shows the main features of a typical human cell.

Components of the Human Cell

Cell Membrane

The cell membrane (plasmalemma) forms the outer boundary of the cell. The selective permeability of the cell membrane allows the cell to interact with its environment in a controlled way. The cell membrane is composed of a fluid combination of lipids (phospholipids and cholesterol), proteins and a small amount of carbohydrates. The basic structure of the cell membrane is formed by a phospholipid bilayer (Figure 1.2). The hydrophilic head region of the phospholipids faces the exterior (extracellular fluid or interstitial or tissue fluid) or aqueous interior (intracellular fluid or cytoplasmic face) of the cell, while the hydrophobic tails remain isolated. A variety of proteins attach to the surface of the phospholipid bilayer, while others traverse it partly or completely. The membrane proteins perform a variety of roles including: *channel proteins*, which facilitate passive transport across the cell membrane;

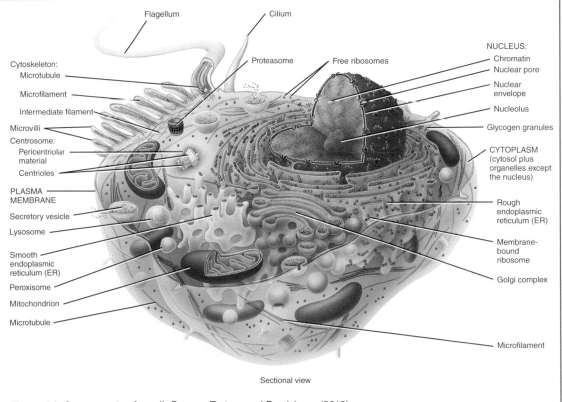

Figure 1.1 Components of a cell. *Source:* Tortora and Derrickson (2013).

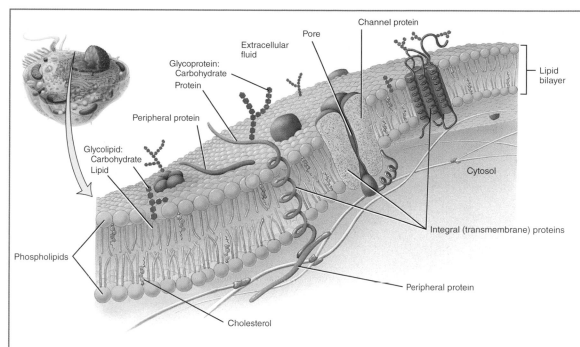

Figure 1.2 Fluid mosaic model of plasma membrane. *Source:* Tortora and Derrickson (2013).

protein pumps for active transport (Chapter 2); and *receptor proteins* for hormones and other endogenous as well as exogenous chemicals. Carbohydrates are either found in combination with proteins (glycoproteins) or lipids (glycolipids) and function as recognition markers, allowing the immune system to differentiate 'self' from foreign cells.

Nucleus

The nucleus is a double membrane-bound structure and measures approximately 3–14 μm in most cells. It stores the DNA and associated proteins (= chromatin) in the form of chromosomes. The nuclear membrane (nucleolemma) isolates the DNA from the cytoplasm and is continuous with the endoplasmic reticulum (Figure 1.1). The nucleolemma contains pores to allow passage of messenger RNA (mRNA) units of nucleic acid. The gel-like portion of the nucleus is known as nucleoplasm. Within the nucleus, proteins, DNA, and ribonucleic acid (RNA) are concentrated around specific chromosomal regions to form the *nucleolus* (plural: nucleoli). The nucleolus itself is not bound by a membrane and is responsible for synthesis of ribosomes.

The functions of the cell are coded in the genes. The genetic code or nucleotide sequence of DNA in the genes is used to direct protein synthesis, a process known as gene expression. First, the DNA is used as a template to link nucleotides, forming a strand of an mRNA molecule. This process is referred to as *transcription* and is facilitated by the enzyme RNA polymerase. The mRNA is then transferred across the nucleolemma into the cytoplasm and is used as a template by ribosomes to synthesise proteins, a process referred to as *translation*. Further processing of the proteins such as addition of phosphate (phosphorylation) or carbohydrates (glycosylation) takes place through a process known as *post-translation modification*.

The nucleus is present in all cells of the body, excluding red blood cells and platelets. Liver cells (hepatocytes) can have one or two nuclei, while the osteoclasts and skeletal muscle cells are multinucleated.

Cytoplasm

The cytoplasm refers to the contents of the cell bounded by the cell membrane on the outer aspect and the nucleus in the inner part of the cell

(Figure 1.1). The liquid portion of the cytoplasm is termed cytosol, and contains mainly water (70–85%), proteins (10–20%), lipids (2%), carbohydrates (1%), and electrolytes. Two distinct components of the cytoplasm include:

- *Organelles*, which are membrane-bound structures with a specific metabolic function. The membrane around different organelles serves to isolate the chemical reactions in the cytoplasm from each other.
- *Inclusions*, which are non-membrane-bound particulate matter in the cytoplasm and do not have any specific metabolic function.

Cytoplasmic Organelles

- *Ribosomes*

Ribosomes are small spherical structures (15 nm in diameter) which may exist as free-floating particles or can be found in clusters lining the outer membrane of the rough endoplasmic reticulum. Ribosomes are the site of protein synthesis and translate the message obtained from the nucleus via transcription and effectively function as the working template or conveyor belt for assembling proteins.

- *Endoplasmic Reticulum*

ER consists of a complex and multi-folded system of parallel membranes and tubules which is contiguous with the nuclear membrane and Golgi apparatus.

The rough endoplasmic reticulum (rER) is studded with ribosomes. rER works with the ribosomes to synthesise proteins which are collected in spaces (cisternae) within the rER. A limited amount of packaging of proteins also takes place in the rER (pancreas).

The smooth endoplasmic reticulum (sER) contributes to lipid metabolism, including synthesis of steroid hormones, the lipid portion of lipoprotein in the liver, and lipid absorption and resynthesis of triglycerides in the intestinal mucosa. sER in skeletal and cardiac muscle, known as the sarcoplasmic reticulum, sequesters calcium for the cytosol. Finally, ER inactivates harmful by-products of metabolism and drugs (liver).

- *Golgi Apparatus*

The Golgi apparatus (GA) like the ER, is also a stacked series of folded membranous sacs. Its main function is to process and package both proteins and non-proteins. The GA is the central delivery system from the cell and 'packages' cellular products into secretory vesicles which bud off from main Golgi membranes to enable them to migrate to and merge with the plasma membrane, releasing their contents outside the cell by a process known as exocytosis. The GA additionally produces lysosomes and digestion-related organelles.

- *Lysosomes*

Lysosomes are small membranous compartments (25–50 nm in diameter) which emanate from the GA. Lysosomes contain several degradative enzymes and assist in the degradation of toxic and waste cell products, including cell debris as well as microbial organisms (e.g. bacteria). Although found in all cells (except erythrocytes), lysosomes are particularly prominent in macrophages and neutrophils. Lysosomes also play a key role in programmed cell death, or *apoptosis*.

- *Peroxisomes*

Peroxisomes are membrane-bound structures, somewhat larger than lysosomes (0.3–1.5 μm in diameter), which arise from ER. They contain specific enzymes (oxidases and catalases) which help the breakdown of long-chain lipids and are involved in the detoxification of certain chemicals (e.g. converting hydrogen peroxide to water). Apart from macrophages, peroxisomes are prominent in liver cells where they are involved in the degradation of alcohol.

- *Secretory Vesicles*

These have a predominantly storage and transport role in cells and originate from the GA. These typically are transported by non-constitutive secretion, which means that the secretions are released continuously regardless of any external factors. This is the standard mechanism and ensures proteins and other important molecules are continuously maintained at the plasma membrane. Non-constitutive transport is very much regulated and requires specific signalling pathways to get the proteins delivered to the cell membrane.

- *Mitochondria*

Mitochondria (singular: mitochondrion) are 0.75–3 μm in diameter and produce energy required for cell functions, effectively functioning as the powerhouse of the cell. They consist of a double-layered membrane. Their inner membrane is highly folded into *cristae*, which markedly increase its surface area. Mitochondria have their own DNA, which allows independent replication of mitochondria and synthesis of enzymes and proteins involved in cellular respiration. They are studded with enzyme-rich proteins responsible for production of energy molecules known as adenosine triphosphate (ATP). Mitochondria use oxygen (cellular respiration) to liberate energy stored in the sugars through a process known as *oxidative phosphorylation*. The energy is stored in the ATP molecules and is used for various cell functions such as protein synthesis and transport. Mitochondria are most numerous in cells with high energy requirements such as the cells in muscle and liver. In addition, mitochondria also store intracellular calcium.

• *Cytoskeletal Components*

The cells are supported by a cytoskeletal network of extensive microtubules and microfilaments and intermediate filaments, which act as a scaffold for cell integrity, provide cell shape as well as being an additional means of transport of substances throughout the cell.

• *Microtubules*

Microtubules are hollow cylindrical structures (25 nm in diameter) and are predominantly made up of α-tubulin and β-tubulin proteins. They have a role in the cellular transport of organelles such as mitochondria and vesicles. They also contribute to the *axoneme*, a cytoskeletal core in cellular appendages like cilia (respiratory tract, fallopian tubes) and flagella (sperms). Finally, microtubules also contribute to centrioles which help in cell division.

• *Intermediate Filaments*

Intermediate filaments are made of fibrous proteins (8–10 nm in diameter) and contribute to the structural integrity and shape of the cell. Examples include: cytokeratin (epithelia, hair, nails); vimentin (connective tissue, blood cells); desmin and synemin (muscle, Z-line proteins); and neurofilaments (neurons).

• *Microfilaments*

Microfilaments are narrow (7 nm) filamentous structures made of the globular protein actin – a very common cell filament (Figure 1.3). They are located near to the inner surface of the cell membrane and help the cell to maintain its shape, and are involved in contraction (muscle) and movement (white blood cells).

Inclusions

Inclusions represent particulate regions in the cytoplasm which are not membrane-bound. These include stored food (e.g. glycogen particles, fat

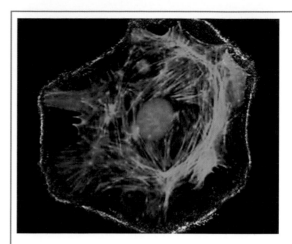

Figure 1.3 A human osteoblast cell stained for actin cytoskeletal filaments (green), plasma cell membrane (orange) and nucleus (blue). Figure courtesy Dr. Vehid Salih

droplets); pigments (melanin, lipofuscin, haemosiderin). Pathological inclusions include bacteria, viruses, and exogenous particulate matter, such as carbon or asbestos in the lungs (not seen in Figure 1.1).

Cell Regeneration and Repair

Cells are said to be in a homeostatic state when they can perform their function normally. However, cells may get damaged from a variety of causes, such as lack of oxygen, physical or chemical agents, nutritional deficiencies, infection, genetic defects, and immunological reactions. Human cells vary in their ability to withstand injury as well as in their ability to regenerate. For example, the cells in the skin and lining mucosae continue to be replaced throughout life while brain and heart cells have limited regenerative ability. Irreversible cell injury results in cell death, which can translate into organ dysfunction, disease, and even death. The dental tissues possess limited capacity for regeneration and repair. The tooth enamel does not contain living cells and cannot regenerate. However, enamel can be remineralised in the early stages of tooth decay prior to cavitation. The dentin-pulp complex and the periodontium, on the other hand, contain living cells (including stem cells) and can undergo regeneration and/or repair to a limited extent, depending on the severity of the injury.

Stem Cells

Stem cells are undifferentiated cells of a multicellular organism which can divide indefinitely to give rise to more cells of the same type (totipotent), and from which certain other types of cell arise by differentiation (multipotent, pluripotent). Stem cells have the capacity therefore to self-renew and to differentiate into different cell types or tissues during embryonic development and typically throughout adulthood, too, although their differentiation potential declines with age. They are classified into two groups based on their origin: *embryonic* stem cells, which are pluripotent and can develop into *any* type of cell, and *adult* stem cells, which are deemed multipotent and these can develop into *many* cell types.

Embryonic stem cells offer immense promise but their clinical use and feasibility are limited, owing to ethical concerns. Adult stem cells may be harvested from different kind of tissues, like bone marrow, umbilical cord, amniotic fluid, brain tissue, liver, pancreas, cornea, various periodontal tissues, and even adipose tissue. Stem cells are currently used in a variety of research applications and for treating diseases of importance (e.g. dementia) as well as debilitating genetic conditions. The role of future stem cell therapy suggests that an adult's own (autologous) cells could be derived, differentiated, and utilised for cell therapy interventions.

Reference

Tortora, G.J. and Derrickson, B. (2013). *Principles of Anatomy and Physiology*. Hoboken, NJ: Wiley.

Further Reading

Hall, J.E. (2015). Chapter 2. In: *Guyton and Hall Textbook of Medical Physiology*, vol. 13. Philadelphia: Elsevier.
Khan Academy (2018). Structure of a cell. https://www.khanacademy.org/science/biology/structure-of-a-cell (accessed 1 May 2018).
Nucleus Medical Media (2018). Biology: Cell structure. https://www.youtube.com/watch?v=URUJD5NEXC8 (accessed 1 May 2018).

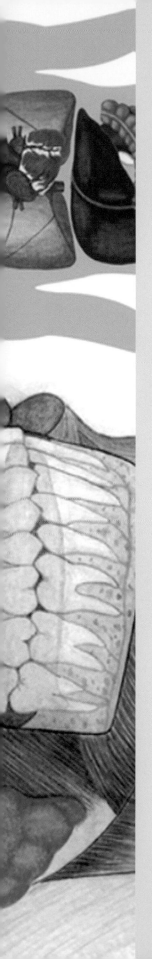

PART II
Nerve Muscle Physiology

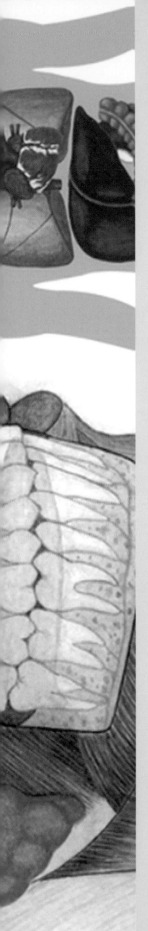

CHAPTER 2
Nerve Physiology

Elizabeth Prabhakar and Kamran Ali

Key Topics

■ Structure and classification of neurons
■ Nerve cell excitability

Learning Objectives

To demonstrate an understanding of the:

■ Distribution of ions in the extracellular and intracellular fluids
■ Role of ion channels in the propagation of nerve impulses
■ Generation and propagation of nerve action potentials
■ Clinical relevance of nerve dysfunction to dental practice

Introduction

Nerves are part of the peripheral nervous system (PNS), consisting of bundles or tracts of nerve fibres (axons) running parallel to each other. The fibres connect the central nervous system (CNS) to the PNS and serve as an important conduit for information flow (in the form of electrical or nerve impulses) between the two systems. Nerves originate from specialised cells called *neurons* which form the basic structural and functional units of the nervous system. The fibres terminate on peripheral target organs, like muscles or glands, called *effectors*. Neurons can be classified functionally into two main types depending on the direction of information flow: (i) sensory (afferent), if impulses are transmitted from the periphery to the CNS and (ii) motor (efferent), if impulses travel from the CNS to the *effectors* in the periphery. Neurons are also categorised structurally as unipolar or multipolar depending on the number of processes (branches) attached to the cell body. The afferent sensory neuron is unipolar because it has one process (axon) attached to its cell body. The efferent motor neuron is multipolar

Essential Physiology for Dental Students, First Edition. Edited by Kamran Ali and Elizabeth Prabhakar.
© 2019 John Wiley & Sons Ltd. Published 2019 by John Wiley & Sons Ltd.
Companion website: www.wiley.com/go/ali/physiology

because it has many processes (dendrites) attached to the cell body (Fig 2.1).

Structure of a Neuron

A neuron consists of three main parts: a cell body or *soma*, dendrites, and an axon. However, the arrangement of these components is different between sensory and motor neurons, as shown in Figure 2.1. In a sensory neuron, dendrites lie distal to the cell body (in the tissues) and consist of a branching network of free nerve endings which transmit nerve impulses towards the CNS (Figure 2.1a). The axon lies mesially and synapses with the nuclei in the CNS to transmit incoming impulses. The cell body in a sensory neuron is interposed between the dendrites and the axon. It provides the metabolic support to the cell but is not involved in impulse transmission. In a motor neuron, the cell body not only provides the metabolic support for the cell but is also involved in impulse transmission from the CNS to the effectors (Figure 2.1b and 2.2).

An axon is a long cylindrical structure representing a single nerve fibre (Figure 2.2). It contains the cytoplasm (axoplasm) enclosed in the nerve membrane (axolemma) which isolates the axoplasm from the surrounding extracellular fluid (ECF). The axolemma consists of a lipid bilayer with the hydrophilic (polar) ends facing the exterior, while the hydrophobic (nonpolar) ends project into the middle of the membrane. Various proteins are associated with the axolemma and include: *transport* proteins (carriers, channels, and pumps) and *receptor* proteins.

In addition to the axolemma, nerve fibres (except the smallest ones) are enclosed in spirally wrapped sheath of lipoprotein known as *myelin*. Concentric layers of myelin are secreted by specialised glial cells, known as *Schwann cells*, which are found in the outermost layer of myelin.

Myelin is absent between adjacent Schwann cells and leads to constrictions, known as *nodes of Ranvier*, on the exterior of the axolemma at regular intervals (every 0.3–0.5 mm). The axolemma is directly exposed to the ECF at the nodes of Ranvier, allowing faster transmission of nerve impulses in large-diameter myelinated nerve fibres. The small diameter unmyelinated nerve fibres are surrounded by nonmyelinating Schwann cells.

A classification of peripheral nerve fibres according to fibre type and properties is depicted in Table 2.1.

The large-diameter A-fibre afferents (myelinated) are involved in conducting impulses from proprioceptors in the muscle and joints to the CNS, while the efferents are involved in muscle contraction and

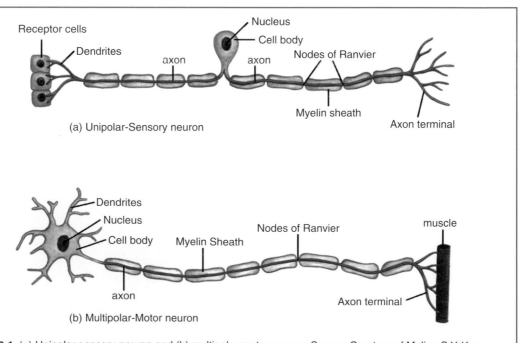

Figure 2.1 (a) Unipolar sensory neuron and (b) multipolar motor neuron. *Source:* Courtesy of Melina S.Y. Kam.

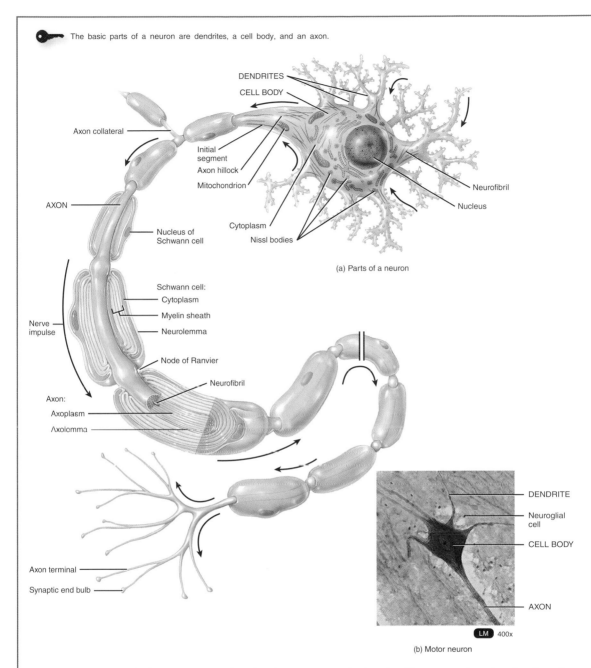

🔑 The basic parts of a neuron are dendrites, a cell body, and an axon.

DENDRITES

CELL BODY

Axon collateral

Initial segment

Axon hillock

Mitochondrion

AXON

Nucleus of Schwann cell

Cytoplasm

Nissl bodies

Neurofibril

Nucleus

(a) Parts of a neuron

Schwann cell:
  Cytoplasm
  Myelin sheath
  Neurolemma

Nerve impulse

Node of Ranvier

Neurofibril

Axon:
  Axoplasm
  Axolemma

Axon terminal

Synaptic end bulb

DENDRITE

Neuroglial cell

CELL BODY

AXON

LM 400x

(b) Motor neuron

Figure 2.2 Typical multipolar motor neuron found at the neuromuscular junction. The arrows show the direction of impulses in an efferent motor neuron. *Source:* Tortora and Derrickson (2017).

aligning joints into the appropriate positions for movement or maintaining muscle tone. The smaller Aδ and C-fibres (unmyelinated) are sensory afferents involved with providing information about pain, touch, and temperature sensations.

The medium-diameter B-fibres and small-diameter C-fibre efferents form part of the autonomic nervous system, which innervate various target organs in the body (Chapter 22). Examples of sensory receptors for touch (Meissner's corpuscle or

Table 2.1 Classification of peripheral nerve fibres.

Type of Fibre	Subclass	Myelin	Diameter (Microns)	Conduction velocity (m s⁻¹)	Location	Function
A	Alpha	+	6–22	30–120	Afferent and efferent from muscles and joints	Motor, Proprioception
	Beta	+	6–22	30–120	Afferent and efferent from muscles and joints	Motor, Proprioception
	Gamma	+	3–6	15–35	Efferent to muscle spindles	Muscle tone
	Delta	+	1–4	5–25	Afferent sensory	Pain, touch, temperature
B		+	< 3	3–15	Preganglionic sympathetic (efferent)	Autonomic
C	sC	–	0.3–1.3	0.7–1.3	Postganglionic sympathetic (efferent)	Autonomic
	d gammaC	–	0.4–1.2	0.1–2.0	Afferent sensory and efferent	Pain, touch, temperature, autonomic

Source: Berde and Strichartz (2000).

Merkel disc), pressure (Pacinian corpuscle), pain (nociceptor) and temperature (thermoreceptor) are shown in Figure 2.3.

Physiology of Peripheral Nerve

Nerve fibres are analogous to electrical cables, in that they transmit electrical impulses (action potentials) to and from the CNS. The impulses are electrical manifestations of the physical and chemical sensations of pain, touch, pressure, temperature, taste, etc. from the PNS to the CNS. Thus, the interconversion of one form of energy (physical/chemical sensations) to another form (electrical impulses) that occurs during information flow is termed *transduction*. Similar transduction processes occur when electrical energy is converted to chemical energy (chemical transmission at the neuromuscular junction) or mechanical energy (muscle contraction or secretions from glands).

The generation and conduction of action potentials depend on the concentrations and permeabilities of two important ions (Na^+ and K^+) moving across the cell membranes of *excitable cells* (nerve and muscle cells or their fibres). The movement of ions is regulated by transport proteins in the cell membrane, called *ion channels*, which in turn have sensors or gates to control entry and exit of ions.

There are three types of types of ion channels involved in the transmission of impulses:

1. Voltage-gated channels (like Na^+, K^+, Ca^{2+}, Cl^-), which *open* if there is a change in membrane potential.
2. Second-messenger gated channels (also called metabotropic), which indirectly control the opening and closing of ion channels, by binding to signalling molecules, like cAMP, IP3, etc.
3. Ligand-gated channels (also called ionotropic channels, which respond to hormones and neurotransmitters). These include the nicotinic acetylcholine receptor on the post synaptic membrane (motor end plate) of the neuromuscular synapse (junction between the cranial nerve and skeletal facial muscle in the orofacial region).

The external surface of the axolemma is surrounded by ECF, while the internal surface is in contact with axoplasm or intracellular fluid (ICF). Both fluid compartments contain a number of solutes (charged and uncharged molecules) dissolved in water. Hence, the chemical composition of the fluid compartments is similar, although the concentration of each solute/ion (mEq l⁻¹) is different

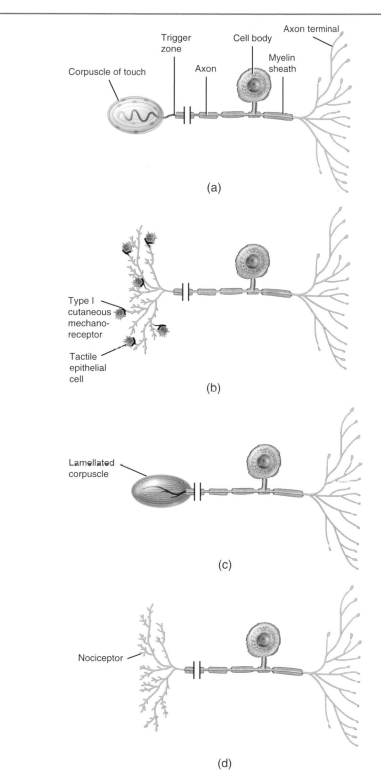

Figure 2.3 Examples of unipolar sensory receptors for touch (a, b), pressure (c), and pain or temperature (d). *Source:* Tortora and Derrickson (2011).

Table 2.2 Chemical composition of extracellular and intracellular fluid compartments.

Solutes (mEq l^{-1})	Extracellular fluid	Intracellular fluid
Na$^+$	140	14
K$^+$	4	120
Ca^{2+}	2.5	1×10^{-4}
Cl$^-$	105	10
HCO^{3-}	24	10
pH	7.4	7.1
Osmolarity	290	290

Source: Adapted from Costanzo (2017).
The anions (negatively charged ions) in intracellular fluid are proteins and organic phosphates.

(Table 2.2). Despite the differences in concentrations of solutes, the total solute concentration (osmolarity) remains the same in the two compartments. This is because water moves freely through the semipermeable cell membrane separating ICF and ECF, bringing the osmolarity to 290 milliosmoles l^{-1} (mOsm l^{-1}) in both compartments. Another interesting feature of the fluid compartments it that they are both electrically neutral, because the concentrations of cations and anions is the same on either side of the cell membrane. With particular regard to the concentrations of Na$^+$ and K$^+$, which are important for action potential generation, it can be seen that the concentration of Na$^+$ is higher outside [Na$^+$]$_o$ in the ECF than on the inside ICF [Na$_+$]$_i$.

The opposite is true for K$^+$, where [K$^+$]$_o$ is low in ECF and [K$^+$]$_i$ and high in ICF. These differences are significant because the concentration gradient across the cell membrane is the main driving force for the movement of an ion. Thus, when ions are transported downhill (from high concentration to low concentration) without the need for energy, the process is called *passive transport* (like diffusion of Na$^+$ and K$^+$ and facilitated diffusion of amino-acids and glucose in many cells of the body). If energy adenosine triphosphate (ATP) is required for the uphill transport (from low concentration to high concentration) then the process is called *active transport* (like primary and secondary active transport, in the renal and intestinal systems and sodium potassium pump in excitable cells). The processes of

facilitated diffusion, primary active transport, and secondary active transport all involve integral membrane proteins which transport molecules. Hence these can also be termed *carrier-mediated transport*.

Contribution of ions in ECF and ICF to resting potential (V$_r$) and equilibrium potential (V$_{eq}$)

Nerve and muscle cells at rest (eg absence of stimulus, like pain) show the distribution of ions in ECF and ICF, as per Table 2.2. This is normally described in terms of concentration gradient or concentration differences of solutes/ions. However, as ions are charged particles, we call this concentration difference a *potential difference* or *resting potential*, denoted by the symbol, V$_r$. The resting potential is also the period between action potentials (evoked in response to a stimulus). The distribution of ions at rest shown in Table 2.2 makes the cell membrane *polarised*.

The V$_r$ is critically dependent on the concentration gradient of the K$^+$ (see below) with approximate values recorded between –70 and –90 mV on the inside of the cell membrane, with respect to the outside, which is positive. The negative value of V$_r$ is partly due to the presence of negatively charged proteins (anions) which are trapped in the ICF, because they are too large to diffuse out of the cell.

As described above, V$_r$ is dependent on concentration gradient of K$^+$, and thus is close to the K$^+$ equilibrium potential (V$_{eq K^+}$). What is the difference between the two potentials, V$_r$ and V$_{eq K^+}$? The value of V$_r$ is influenced by the ion species with the greatest permeability (often described as *conductance*) at rest i.e. K$^+$. Thus, K$^+$ diffuses easily through ion or 'leak' channels which are fully open at rest, allowing outward downhill diffusion of K$^+$. Thus, loss of cations or positively charged K$^+$ leaves behind more negatively charged anions inside the membrane, making V$_r$ negative. In comparison, Na$^+$ permeability is low at rest and so V$_r$ is far away from V$_{eq Na^+}$. Hence V$_r$ can only be as negative as V$_{eq K^+}$. But how? To explain this, we need to remember that equilibrium potential, electrochemical equilibrium or reversal potential for K$^+$ can be described as the membrane potential (V$_m$) at which the net flow through any open K$^+$ channel is 0. In other words, the chemical (concentration of ion) and electrical (charge on the permeant ion) are in balance. This electrochemical or equilibrium potential for each ion species can be calculated using the Nernst equation. Using this equation, the $V_{eq\ K^+}$ is approximately –88 mV and that of $V_{eq\ Na^+}$ is approximately +60 mV. Thus, the measured V_r which is approximately –90 mV is close to the calculated equilibrium potential of K⁺ of –88 mV.

The resting potential is maintained by the action of the electrogenic Na⁺-K⁺-ATPase pump, which actively extrudes 3Na⁺ ions for every 2K⁺ ions transported simultaneously into the cell.

Inhibition of the electrogenic pump by drugs like ouabain and digitalis (cardiac glycosides) will cause intracellular accumulation of Na⁺ or a corresponding decrease in K⁺. Such an inhibition would disrupt the concentration gradient of each ion, and the upstroke of the action potential would be prevented, leaving the person unable to respond to any stimulus, which could be fatal.

A deviation from the resting potential will give rise to action potential, involving voltage-gated Na⁺ and K⁺ ion channels in the cell membrane, as described earlier. The events are summarised in Figure 2.4a and b.

1. *Rest:* All voltage-gated Na⁺ and K⁺ channels are closed (but leak channels are still open, allowing K⁺ to diffuse out of the cell. The voltage-gated Na⁺ channel has two gates: the activation gate and the inactivation gate. In the resting state, the activation gate is closed but the inactivation gate is open, making it impossible for Na⁺ to enter the cell. The voltage-gated K⁺ channel, on the other hand, only has one gate, which is closed, at rest, 70 mV.
2. *Depolarisation:* When a stimulus like pain or taste is perceived by the appropriate sensory receptor, an electrical disturbance occurs across its cell membrane, depolarising the membrane from its earlier resting 'polarised' state. This causes an increase in Na⁺ permeability and makes the inside of the cell membrane less negative or more positive. This causes both activation and inactivation gates of the voltage-gated Na⁺ channel to open (note that the inactivation gate was already open in the resting state), allowing diffusion of Na⁺ into the cell. A small inward Na⁺ current is produced, which further depolarises the cell membrane. When the depolarisation reaches a critical threshold around –55 mV, more activation gates open to allow further influx of Na⁺ via positive feedback, until all activation gates are open. At this point,

the permeability of Na⁺ is 1000 times greater than it was at rest. The V_m overshoots to +30 mV (but does not quite reach the Na⁺ equilibrium potential of +60 mV). This is the upstroke of the action potential. Local anaesthetics like lidocaine offer pain control by blocking voltage-gated Na⁺ channels in a reversible manner to prevent action potentials. Similar effects are produced by Tetrodotoxin (a toxin from the Japanese puffer fish). This means the person will be unable to respond to a pain stimulus while under dental treatment.

3. *Repolarisation:* The Na⁺ activation gates close rapidly. As the V_m reaches 0 mV, the slower Na⁺ inactivation gates begin to close, while voltage-sensitive K⁺ gates open. The permeability of Na⁺ (P_{Na^+}) decreases, thus terminating the upstroke of action potential, in ~1 ms. The opening of K⁺ channels causes an increased permeability of K⁺ (P_{K^+}), causing an efflux of K⁺ out of the cell. The combination of closing Na⁺ inactivation channels and opening K⁺ channels makes the K⁺ conductance much higher than the Na⁺ conductance, giving rise to an outward K⁺ current. This repolarising of the membrane causes the downward deflection (downstroke) of the action potential. The chemical tetraethylammonium (TEA) blocks voltage-gated K⁺ channels and thus the outward K⁺ current.
4. *Hyperpolarisation (or afterpotential or undershoot):* Owing to the high P_{K^+} and slow closure of voltage-gated K⁺ channels, there is a continuous efflux of K⁺ for a short time following repolarisation. The efflux exceeds that seen at rest and undershoots (goes beyond) resting potential of –70 mV, reaching a value of –88 mV, therefore called *after-hyperpolarising phase* (Figure 2.4b). The afterpotential approximates the K⁺ equilibrium potential. When all K⁺ channels close, the cell membrane returns to the resting level. The membrane may be ready to generate another action potential if a stimulus is applied and the cell is not in the 'absolute refractory period'.

Refractory Period

The refractory period is that time period when the cell is unable to fire another action potential irrespective of the strength of the stimulus. This is

(a)

Inflow of sodium ions (na⁺) causes the depolarising phase, and outflow of potassium ions (K⁺) causes the repolarising phase of an action potential.

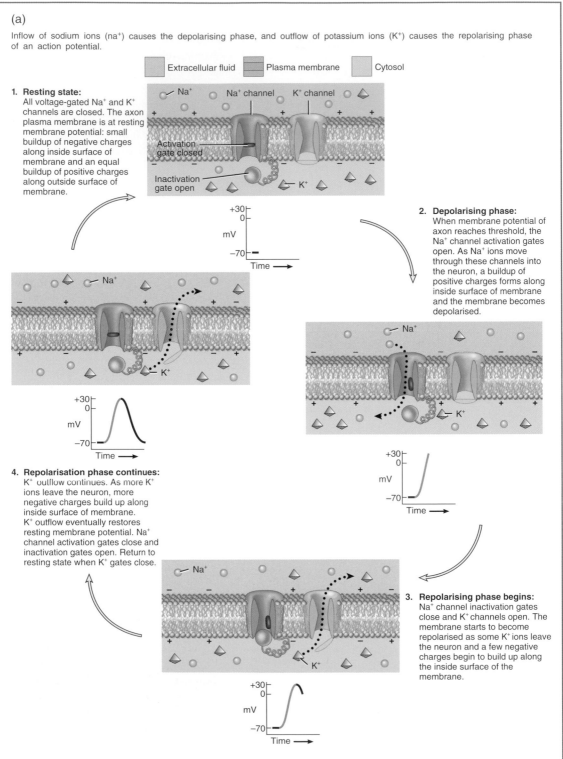

1. Resting state:
All voltage-gated Na⁺ and K⁺ channels are closed. The axon plasma membrane is at resting membrane potential: small buildup of negative charges along inside surface of membrane and an equal buildup of positive charges along outside surface of membrane.

2. Depolarising phase:
When membrane potential of axon reaches threshold, the Na⁺ channel activation gates open. As Na⁺ ions move through these channels into the neuron, a buildup of positive charges forms along inside surface of membrane and the membrane becomes depolarised.

4. Repolarisation phase continues:
K⁺ outflow continues. As more K⁺ ions leave the neuron, more negative charges build up along inside surface of membrane. K⁺ outflow eventually restores resting membrane potential. Na⁺ channel activation gates close and inactivation gates open. Return to resting state when K⁺ gates close.

3. Repolarising phase begins:
Na⁺ channel inactivation gates close and K⁺ channels open. The membrane starts to become repolarised as some K⁺ ions leave the neuron and a few negative charges begin to build up along the inside surface of the membrane.

Figure 2.4 (a) Changes in ion flow through voltage-gated channels during the depolarising and repolarising phases of an action potential. Leak channels and sodium–potassium pumps are not shown. *Source:* Tortora and Derrickson (2017).

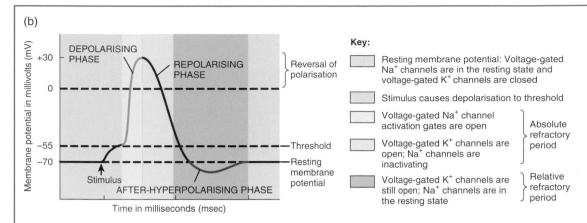

Figure 2.4 (Continued) (b) Action potential or impulse. The action potential arises at the trigger zone (here, at the junction of the axon hillock and the initial segment) of the neuronal cell body, which propagates along the axon to the axon terminals. The green and yellow regions of the neuron indicate parts that typically have voltage-gated Na^+ and K^+ channels (axolemma and axon terminals). *Source:* Tortora and Derrickson (2017).

called the *absolute refractory period*. The absolute refractory period is usually between 0 and 3 ms. This is because depolarisation causes all Na^+ inactivation gates to close until repolarisation is complete. The time period following repolarisation, approximately between 3 and 4 ms, is called the *relative refractory period*, which overlaps with hyperpolarisation (Figure 2.4b). During this time, an action potential can be evoked, but only with a very intense stimulus. The strong stimulus will cause the rapid opening of Na^+ activation gates and the firing of an action potential.

Generally, however, if an intense stimulus is not applied, the relative refractory period ensures that each action potential is a separate 'all or none' phenomenon.

This is because, the negative 'undershoot' is further away from the resting potential, making it difficult for the cell membrane to reach the 'threshold' of -55 mV and firing an action potential.

Clinical Relevance

Individuals with high serum K^+ levels are unable to elicit action potentials in response to a stimulus. In patients with hyperkalaemia, a phenomenon known as *accommodation* is seen. This is when the threshold potential is bypassed, owing to the closure of Na^+ inactivation gates that normally open during depolarisation. Thus, the increased serum (extracellular) K^+ concentration would result in diffusion of K^+

into the cell down its concentration gradient. This would make the inside of the cell membrane positive, leading to depolarisation and a subsequent firing of an action potential. However, this does not happen, because sustained depolarisation, paradoxically, closes Na^+ inactivation gates, preventing an action potential (similar to the absolute refractory period). This results in muscular weakness due to inability of muscles to contract

Transmission and Speed of nerve impulses

In peripheral nerves, the impulses can travel rapidly to great distances, along the entire length of an axon, often > 1 metre long. The chemical events involved in propagation of the nerve impulse are similar to those discussed in Fig 2.4a, but with some differences summarised in Fig 2.5. The figure also compares the speed of transmission between an unmyelinated axon (Fig 2.5a, continuous conduction) and myelinated axon (Fig 2.5b, saltatory conduction) at 1 msec, 5 msec and 10 msec intervals.

The events in impulse propagation are initiated in the axon hillock or trigger zone of neuronal cell body in both unmyelinated and myelinated axons, at 1 msec. The stimulus depolarises the trigger zone causing a flow of Na^+ through voltage-gated channels to produce an inward flow of positive current through the axoplasm (the intracellular surface). Simultaneously, positive charges on the outside (extracellular face) of the axon flow back towards the depolarised trigger zone setting up a local circuit (insets in Figure 2.5). As the positive ions move down their concentration gradients within the axoplasm, the local current spreads to the next "inactive" region of the axon and is conducted along the length of axon without interruption. This is called continuous conduction in an unmyelinated axon and can be seen at 5 and 10msec.

Local currents alone would be unable to propagate the action potential because energy would be lost along the way, thus preventing the firing of an action potential. However, this does not happen. Why? Because large fibre axons are myelinated and when localised currents reach voltage-gated Na^+ channels in the Nodes of Ranvier, depolarisation would occur, increasing permeability of Na^+. The influx of Na^+ into the axoplasm, would make the interior of the axolemma positive and evoke an action potential in the active regions (at the nodes where Na^+ enters) of the axon.

Consequently, the increased concentration of Na^+ in the "active region" would cause a local current to spread and depolarise the next "inactive region" further along the axon. This cycle would repeat itself thus propagating the action potential down to the axon terminals. Note that the action potential is only evoked at the Nodes of Ranvier. The magnitude (amplitude) of the action potential remains constant, from start (trigger zone) to finish (axon terminals). In the meantime, the axonal membrane behind the active zone would become refractory, to prevent backward conduction of the action potential. In the active region, K^+ diffuses out of the axoplasm, thereby repolarising the axon.

The distance travelled by an impulse in a myelinated axon is much greater than the distance travelled in an unmyelinated axon at 5msec and 10msec (Fig 2.5).

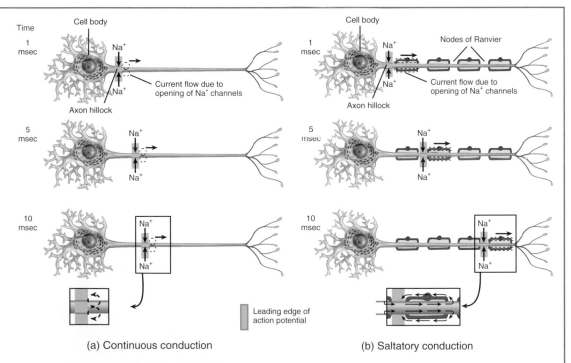

Figure 2.5 Propagation of action potential in a neuron. Dotted lines indicate ionic current flow along the direction of the arrow. The insets show local current circuits. (a) In continuous conduction, along an unmyelinated axon, ionic currents flow across each adjacent segment of the membrane. (b) In saltatory conduction, along a myelinated axon, the action potential (nerve impulse) at the first node of Ranvier generates ionic currents in the cytosol and interstitial fluid that open voltage-gated Na^+ channels in the axolemma at the second node, and so on at each subsequent node. Thus action potential jumps from node to node. *Source:* Tortora and Derrickson (2017).

In myelinated axons, the action potential "jumps" from node to node increasing the rate of impulse conduction. This phenomenon is called *saltatory conduction* (Fig 2.5b) Action potentials are evoked at the nodes, due to the availability of a large number of Na⁺ and K⁺ voltage gated channels. Additionally, the node of Ranvier exhibits low resistance to current flow due to its lack of myelination, which would otherwise impede impulse generation. This is because the fatty myelin sheath, acts as an electrical insulator to increase membrane resistance (and decreases membrane capacitance) on the outside of the axon making it difficult to depolarise the membrane and fire an action potential.

The presence of myelin is also beneficial because its insulating properties protect the axon from the spread of electrical current to unintended target cells.

Clinical Relevance

Local anaesthetic drugs are used to achieve pain control during a variety of dental operative procedures. Administration of local anaesthetics via dental injections causes a reversible blockage of sodium channels in the nerve membrane in the tissues at the injection site. This leads to impairment of nerve impulse conduction, thereby providing adequate pain control (analgesia) allowing a painless dental treatment.

Neuralgia is a pain emanating from a nerve. The commonest neuralgia affecting the face and oral cavity is *trigeminal neuralgia*. It is characterised by severe, sharp electric and shooting pain in the distribution of the trigeminal nerve. The pain is paroxysmal and occurs in bouts lasting for a few seconds to a few minutes. Although it may not have an identifiable cause, it may result from compression of the trigeminal ganglion in the brain by an aberrant blood vessel. Neuralgic pain is caused by rapidly firing neurons and does not respond to routine pain killers. Neuralgia is often managed by membrane-stabilising medications which selectively block nerve impulse conduction in rapidly firing neurons.

Multiple sclerosis is a demyelinating disease affecting the CNS. It may result from immune destruction of the myelin-producing cells. Lack of myelin impairs nerve impulse conduction leading to a variety of sensory, motor, visual, and autonomic deficits. In addition, patients of multiple sclerosis may also present with features of trigeminal neuralgia.

References

Berde, C.B. and Strichartz, G.R. (2000). Local anaesthetics. In: *Anaesthesia*, 5e (ed. R.D. Miller), 491–521. Philadelphia: Churchill Livingstone.

Costanzo, L. (2017). *Neurophysiology in Physiology*, 6e, 65–112. Philadelphia: Elsevier.

Tortora, G.J. and Derrickson, B. (2011). The nervous tissue. In: *Principles of Anatomy and Physiology*, 13e. Wiley.

Tortora, G.J. and Derrickson, B. (2017). The nervous system In: *Principles of Anatomy and Physiology*, 15e. Wiley.

Further Reading

Silverthorn, D.U. (2017). Neurons: Cellular and network properties. In: *Human Physiology: An Integrated Approach*, 7e, 250–295. Pearson Education.

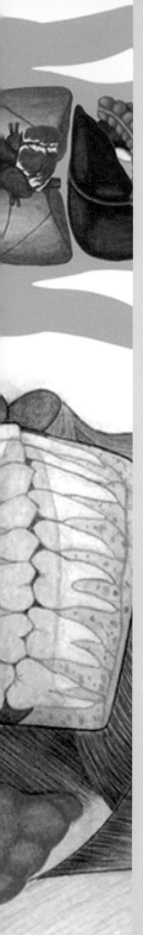

CHAPTER 3
Muscle Physiology

Elizabeth Prabhakar and Kamran Ali

Key Topics

- Structure and classification of muscles
- Organisation and functions of muscle tissue

Learning Objectives

To demonstrate an understanding of the:

- Microscopic structure of skeletal and smooth muscles
- Mechanisms of muscle contraction
- Organisation and functions of the neuromuscular junction
- Common muscle disorders relevant to dental practice

Introduction

Locomotion in living organisms is achieved by specialised cells called skeletal muscles which have the unique ability to *contract* and propel the organism forwards (and in many other directions). Much like the nerve cell, the muscle cell is also capable of *excitability* through the generation of muscle action potentials (triggered by nerve stimulation with the exception of the cardiac muscle). Other properties of the muscle tissue are: *extensibility*, which allows muscles to stretch within limits without causing damage, and *elasticity*, which allows muscles to recoil and return to resting length after a period of stretch.

Types of Muscle

There are three types of muscle: *skeletal*, *cardiac*, and *smooth* (Figure 3.1). The skeletal muscles are under voluntary control and are responsible for movements and stabilisation of the body. They also act as metabolic organs and contribute to heat generation.

Essential Physiology for Dental Students, First Edition. Edited by Kamran Ali and Elizabeth Prabhakar.
© 2019 John Wiley & Sons Ltd. Published 2019 by John Wiley & Sons Ltd.
Companion website: www.wiley.com/go/ali/physiology

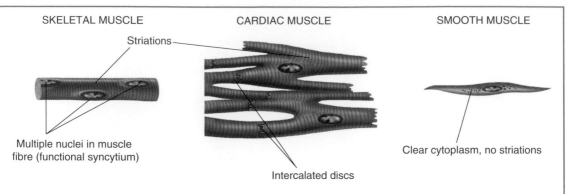

Figure 3.1 Structure of different muscle types: skeletal, cardiac, and smooth muscle. *Source:* Tortora and Derrickson (2017).

In addition, they also protect the internal organs. The cardiac muscle (myocardium) is involuntary in nature (Chapter 4). Smooth muscles are also involuntary and are found in hollow organs like blood vessels and visceral organs such as the gastrointestinal tract (GIT), where they regulate blood flow and help in digestion respectively. Under the microscope, skeletal and cardiac muscles appear striated or striped, while the smooth muscle shows no striations.

Anatomical Organisation of the Skeletal Muscle

A skeletal muscle is so called because it is attached to the bones of the skeleton by tough fibrous connective tissue called *tendons* (Figure 3.2), which confer the properties of flexibility and extensibility. The organisation of all three muscle types is similar. A transverse section through the muscle (Figure 3.2) shows that the muscle is surrounded by a layer of connective tissue (fascia) called *epimysium*. The largest muscle is divided into a number of discrete bundles called *fascicles*. Each fascicle is also surrounded by a layer of connective tissue called *perimysium*. Each fascicle is made up of a number of *muscle fibres* which are enclosed by connective tissue called *endomysium*. Each muscle fibre, in turn, is composed of thinner myofibrils. Each myofibril is made up of myofilaments.

Microscopic Organisation of the Skeletal Muscle

Each muscle fibre is a multinucleate, functional *syncytium* (Figures 3.1 and 3.3) arising from the fusion of smaller mesodermal cells. Such an arrangement makes it possible for the muscle fibre to contract as a single unit and generate the necessary force required to lift heavy objects or generate speed and endurance for athletic events.

Each muscle cell is surrounded by a cell membrane known as *sarcolemma*, which invaginates into the cell to form transverse or T-tubules. These tubules are the microanatomical structures responsible, for the spread of muscle action potentials and further depolarisation (Figure 3.3). As muscle cells are metabolically active, they contain a rich store of glycogen and myoglobin in their sarcoplasm for the production of ATP (adenosine triphosphate) necessary for muscle contraction.

The muscle cell cytoplasm is known as *sarcoplasm* and contains numerous myofibrils, surrounded by the sarcoplasmic reticulum (endoplasmic reticulum), which sequesters Ca^{2+} necessary to initiate muscle contraction. These myofibrils are arranged into discrete units called *sarcomeres*, bounded by Z-lines to demarcate adjacent sarcomeres (Figure 3.4). The sarcomere forms the basic contractile unit and shows a characteristic 'banding' pattern of 'light' and 'dark' bands, containing the contractile proteins actin and myosin, respectively. These bands appear as striations under the microscope in the cardiac and skeletal muscle (Figure 3.1). The dark or A-bands are made up of thick myofilaments, containing myosin. The light or I-bands are composed of thin myofilaments, containing the actin, located on either side of the A-band. Thin myofilaments are attached to Z-lines which course through the centre of each I-band and form the boundaries of a single muscle cell or sarcomere on either side.

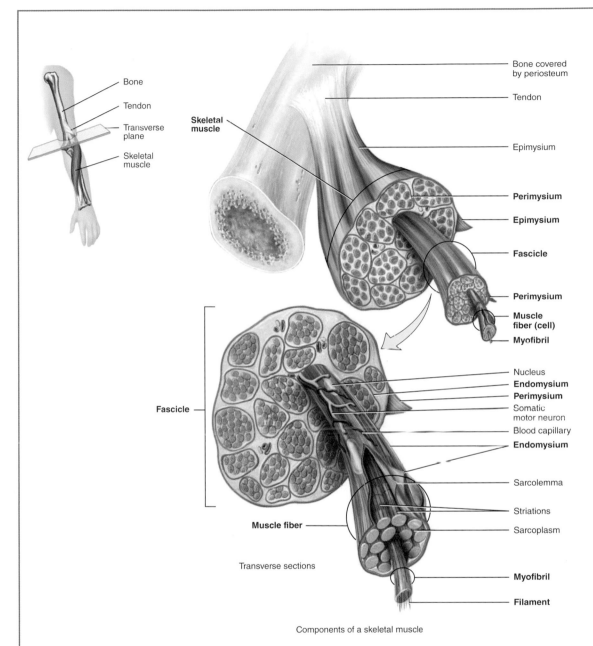

Components of a skeletal muscle

Figure 3.2 Organisation and structure of the skeletal muscle. Tendons attach the skeletal muscle to the bone. The muscle organ is divided into numerous bundles called *fascicles*. Each fascicle consists of a number of muscle fibres (or cells), which in turn contain many myofibrils, made up of thinner myofilaments. Each component of the skeletal muscle is covered by its own outer layer of connective tissue: the epimysium, perimysium, and endomysium respectively. *Source:* Tortora and Derrickson (2017).

Muscle cells are designed to contract. This happens when the Z-lines pull the thin actin myofilaments inwards, to overlap with the thick myosin myofilaments, towards the A-band, thus shortening the muscle fibre (Figure 3.4). Another region, the H-zone, is situated in the centre of the A-band of each sarcomere and does not contain any thin filaments, making it easy for overlap or cross-bridge

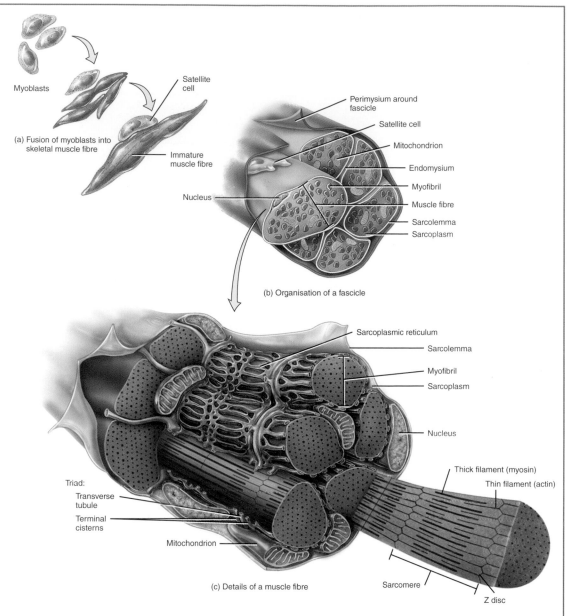

Myoblasts

Satellite cell

(a) Fusion of myoblasts into skeletal muscle fibre

Immature muscle fibre

Nucleus

Perimysium around fascicle

Satellite cell

Mitochondrion

Endomysium

Myofibril

Muscle fibre

Sarcolemma

Sarcoplasm

(b) Organisation of a fascicle

Sarcoplasmic reticulum

Sarcolemma

Myofibril

Sarcoplasm

Nucleus

Thick filament (myosin)

Thin filament (actin)

Triad:
Transverse tubule
Terminal cisterns
Mitochondrion

(c) Details of a muscle fibre

Sarcomere

Z disc

Figure 3.3 Microscopic organisation of skeletal muscle. Muscles arise from the fusion of myoblasts. The sarcolemma or muscle cell membrane has numerous folds which form a system of transverse tubules or T-tubules, through which the rapid transmission of muscle action potentials takes place. *Source:* Tortora and Derrickson (2017).

formation during muscle contraction. The thick myosin filaments are connected together at the M-line in the middle of the A-band. All sarcomeres throughout the entire length of the muscle fibre contract simultaneously to shorten the fibres. This is called the *sliding filament mechanism*, which is discussed later in the chapter.

Structure of Contractile and Regulatory Proteins

Myosin and actin are contractile proteins. The thick myofilament protein, myosin has a 'globular head' and a long 'tail' (Figure 3.5a). The myosin head embeds an actin-binding site and an ATPase-binding

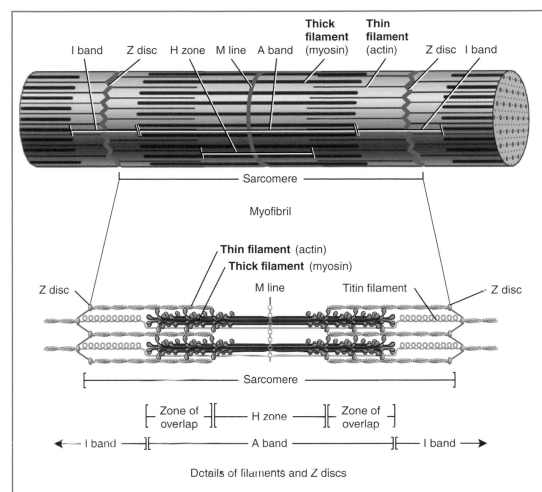

Figure 3.4 Ultrastructure of the muscle fibre, showing light (I) and dark (A) banding patterns, giving the muscle a striated appearance. The bands contain contractile proteins. The I-bands contain the thin actin myofilament and the A-bands contain the thick myofilament. *Source:* Tortora and Derrickson (2017).

site (the site where ATP hydrolysis occurs). Both these sites help with cross-bridge formation during muscle contraction. Thin myofilaments are made up of three different proteins: actin (the contractile protein) and the two regulatory proteins tropomyosin and troponin. Actin is a globular protein and has two myosin-binding sites. At rest, tropomyosin blocks the myosin-binding sites thus preventing cross-bridge formation and muscle contraction (Figure 3.5b). The third protein, troponin, is a complex of three proteins: T, I, and C, which are located at intervals along the tropomyosin filaments. Troponin-T is necessary for attaching the troponin complex to tropomyosin. Troponin-I (in conjunction with tropomyosin) inhibits binding between actin and myosin by blocking myosin-binding site on actin. Troponin-C binds to Ca^{2+} to initiate muscle contraction.

Cytoskeletal or Structural Proteins

Structural proteins, like titin and dystrophin, are present in the muscle cells (Figure 3.4 only shows the protein titin). Titin is the largest protein. It is highly elastic in nature and extends from the M-line along the length of the myosin myofilaments to Z-discs on either side. Titin helps with elastic recoil of a stretched muscle and also in complex signalling pathways in response to weight lifting. The function of cytoskeletal proteins is to maintain sarcomere stability and also to anchor sarcomeres of adjacent myofibrils together.

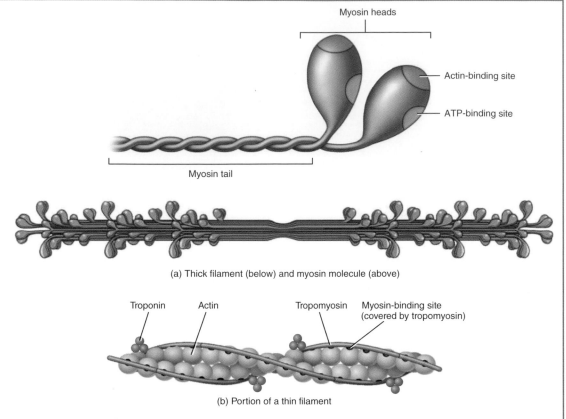

Myosin heads

Actin-binding site

ATP-binding site

Myosin tail

(a) Thick filament (below) and myosin molecule (above)

Troponin   Actin   Tropomyosin   Myosin-binding site
(covered by tropomyosin)

(b) Portion of a thin filament

Figure 3.5 Structure of contractile proteins (a) myosin, thick myofilament with the two binding sites, one for actin and the other for ATPase (b) actin, thin myofilament with two binding sites for myosin. At rest the myosin-binding sites are blocked by the regulatory protein tropomyosin which forms a complex with troponin to prevent cross-bridge formation and thus muscle contraction. *Source:* Tortora and Derrickson (2017).

This whole myofibrillar array is attached to the sarcolemma by another important protein called *dystrophin*. Individuals with no dystrophin or a faulty dystrophin will have muscular dystrophy, leading to weakness and loss of architecture of skeletal muscle mass.

Contraction of the Muscle

Mechanical Aspects

The contraction and relaxation states of the muscle are illustrated in Figure 3.6. Notice how the length of the muscle shortens in the contracted state with corresponding changes in the width of the different bands (discussed below).

Muscle contraction takes place when the actin filaments on both sides move inwards towards the

M-line, sliding past the stationary myosin filaments (overlap) pulling the Z-discs along with them and shortening the length of the muscle fibres. The contraction decreases the width of the H-zone and I-band. The actual width of the A-band and the length of myosin filaments remain the same.

Molecular Aspects: The Sliding Filament Mechanism

At rest, the muscle fibre is unable to contract because the myosin and actin myofilaments cannot bind to form a cross-bridge. This inability to form a cross-bridge is because the myosin-binding sites on the thin actin myofilaments are blocked by the troponin I-tropomyosin complex.

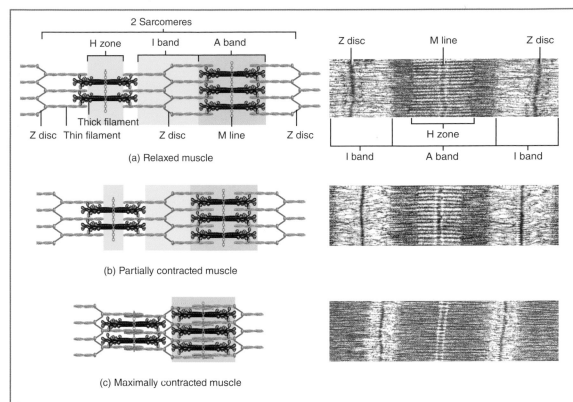

Figure 3.6 Sliding filament model of muscle contraction. (a) Relaxed muscle with no overlap between actin and myosin. Muscle fibre at rest and not contracted. (b) Partially contracted muscle, with some degree of overlap between thick and thin myofilaments. Length of muscle cell is slightly shorter than at rest. (c) Maximally contracted muscle, with actin filaments from both sides fully overlapping myosin. The length of muscle shortened considerably, owing to inward movement of Z-discs being pulled inwards by the actin filaments to which they are attached. The widths of I-band and H-zone have decreased. *Source:* Tortora and Derrickson (2017).

However, when a muscle fibre is depolarised by a nerve action potential, Ca^{2+} is released from the sarcoplasmic reticulum, which binds to troponin C. This binding moves the troponin I-tropomyosin complex out of the way to uncover the myosin-binding site on the actin molecule for cross-bridge formation.

Figure 3.7 shows the sequence of events involved in the sliding filament mechanism.

1. At rest the myosin is said to be in an energised position. This means that an ATP molecule is hydrolysed into $ADP + P_i$ (adenosine diphosphate and inorganic phosphate) at the ATPase-binding site in the myosin head. The ADP and P_i remain attached to the myosin head, putting it in a 90° or cocked position (stored potential energy).

2. Myosin binds to its binding site on the actin myofilament to form a cross-bridge to release the P_i.

3. The cross-bridge or myosin head swivels to 45° (power stroke) pulling the thin actin myofilament along with the Z-line inwards to the M-line or centre of the sarcomere as described earlier. This movement is analogous to the rowing action of a boat, which releases the ADP from the myosin head.

4. A fresh molecule of ATP binds to the myosin head to detach it from the cross-bridge.

If no ATP is available, then the myosin head remains attached to the actin myofilament and *rigour mortis* (stiffness) sets in, as seen in death, i.e. the muscles are in a permanent state of contraction.

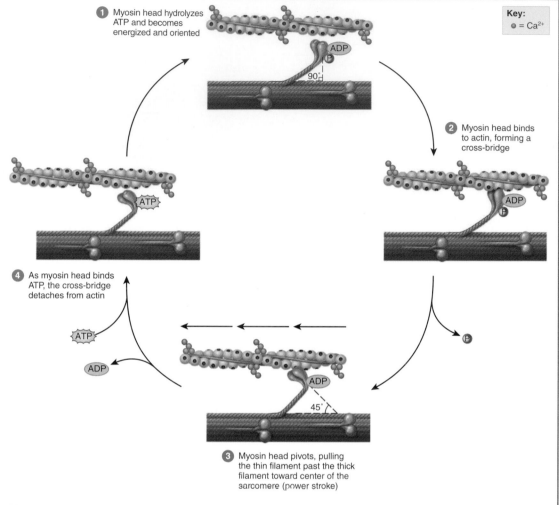

Figure 3.7 The Sliding filament mechanism. Describes the contraction cycle of the skeletal muscle. *Source:* Tortora and Derrickson (2017).

In the living muscle, rigour lasts for a very brief period.

Muscle Relaxation

This takes place when Ca^{2+} is removed and returned to the sarcoplasmic reticulum. This allows tropomyosin to slide back and block the actin-binding site. As the cross-bridge releases, the elastic fibres in the sarcomere recoil, returning the muscle to its original length or resting state.

Since a skeletal muscle can only contract when stimulated by a nerve impulse (termed *neurogenic*), we need to understand the sequence of events which occur at the *synapse* (the junction between the nerve and muscle, also called the *neuromuscular junction*, or NMJ) and couple this to the subsequent process of muscle contraction (the sliding filament mechanism). The entire process is called *excitation-contraction or E-C coupling* in the skeletal muscle.

Neuromuscular Junction (NMJ)

The best-studied example of synaptic transmission is the NMJ. The NMJ is a specialised chemical synapse found in the periphery. The structure of the NMJ (depicted in Figure 3.8) shows the axon collateral of a somatic motor neuron. A single motor

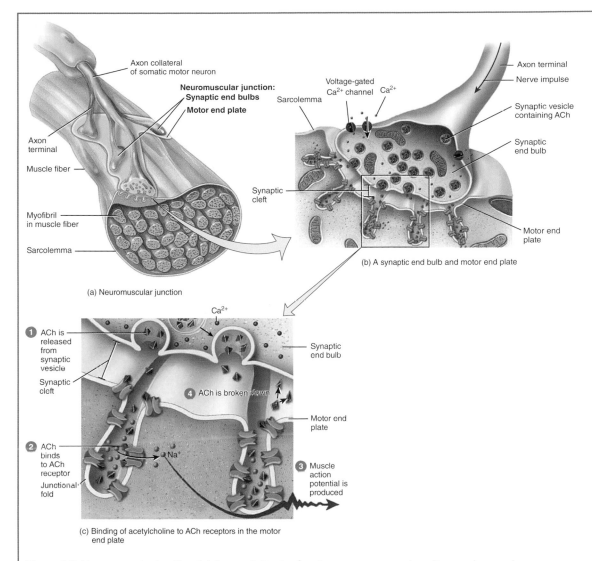

Figure 3.8 Neuromuscular junction. (a) Axon collaterals of motor neurons synapsing with muscle sarcolemma; (b) the arrival of a nerve impulse causes neurotransmitter ACh release into synaptic cleft; (c) binding of ACh to its specific receptor giving rise to muscle action potential. Also shows the breakdown of ACh to prevent further muscle depolarisation which would lead to sustained muscle contraction. *Source:* Tortora and Derrickson (2017).

neuron can innervate multiple muscle fibres, thereby causing the fibres to contract at the same time. The axon collateral has numerous enlarged endings called *synaptic bulbs* (or boutons). These contain secretory vesicles filled with the neurotransmitter acetylcholine (ACh). The area of the muscle fibre opposite the synaptic boutons is called the *motor end plate* and has approximately 40 million ACh receptors.

Excitation-Contraction (E-C) Coupling in a Skeletal Muscle

At the NMJ, a nerve action potential will generate a muscle action potential (Figures 3.8 and 3.9) as follows:

Arrival of nerve action potential releases ACh: An action potential transmitted along the axon collateral of the facial nerve will trigger the opening

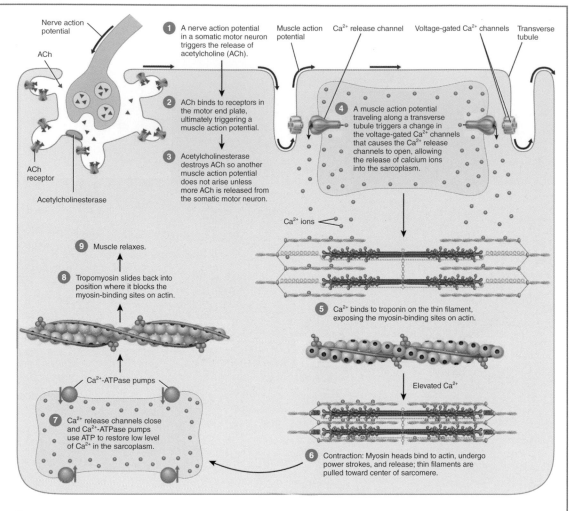

Figure 3.9 Summary of events in the excitation-contraction mechanism of skeletal muscle fibre. *Source:* Tortora and Derrickson (2017).

of voltage-gated Ca^{2+} channels in the presynaptic membrane (Figure 3.8a). This will cause an influx of Ca^{2+} from ECF into the axon terminals down its concentration gradient. Entry of Ca^{2+} stimulates the secretory vesicles in the synaptic bulbs to release ACh into the synaptic cleft via exocytosis (Figure 3.8b). ACh diffuses across the synaptic cleft towards the motor end plate (Figure 3.8c and Figure 3.9, step 1) of the buccinator muscle fibres, for example.

Activation of ACh receptors in postsynaptic cell (motor end plate of the sarcolemma): The ACh molecules released into the synaptic cleft bind to the acetylcholine receptor (AChR) in the sarcolemma (Figures 3.8c and 3.9, step 2). AChR is a ligand-gated channel, which requires the binding of two

ACh molecules (ligands) to activate it. When activation occurs, it triggers the opening of the Na^+ ion channel enclosed within its receptor complex and allows passive diffusion of Na^+ into the muscle cell, down its concentration gradient (this is a typical description of synaptic transmission similar to that which occurs in the central nervous system). Na^+ depolarises sarcolemma.

Depolarisation of muscle cell membrane and muscle action potential: Meanwhile, depolarisation of the sarcolemma elicits a muscle action potential which is propagated through the system of T-tubules. The muscle action potential triggers the release of intracellular Ca^{2+} from sarcoplasmic reticulum into the sarcoplasm (Figure 3.9, step 4). Ca^{2+} combines with troponin to initiate muscle contraction, as described under sliding filament mechanism (Figure 3.9, step 5–9).

Degradation, reuptake, and resynthesis of ACh: In order to prevent further muscle depolarisation and second muscle action potential, ACh must be rapidly hydrolysed into its components, acetyl and choline, by the enzymatic action of acetylcholinesterase (AChE) in the synaptic cleft (Figure 3.9, step 3). These components are unable to activate the ACh receptor and so there is no further depolarisation and contraction. However, as both acetyl and choline are useful products, they are transported back into the synaptic boutons, where they recombine to form ACh. The synthesis of ACh is catalysed by another enzyme, *choline acetyltransferase* (CHAT).

The coordinated muscle contraction involving groups of muscle fibres can be achieved in a synchronised manner, owing to the central location of the NMJ in the muscle fibres. This allows muscle action potentials to be propagated towards both ends of the fibre, causing simultaneous contraction of the fibres in the fascicle.

Smooth Muscle

These muscles are unlike the skeletal and cardiac muscles, as they do not have striations. Although smooth muscles possess thick and thin myofilaments, these are not organised into sarcomeres, with the characteristic light and dark bands. Smooth muscles are involuntary.

Smooth muscles are found in the walls of many hollow organs, like the bladder, uterus, vas deferens, GIT, blood vessels, respiratory airways, eyes, and skin. In the eyes, smooth muscle alters the size of the iris and shape of the lens. In the skin, it causes piloerection. The other functions of smooth muscle are *motility* and maintenance of *tension*. For example, in the GIT, chyme is pushed along by wave-like movements and in the bladder, urine is propelled along the ureters. Smooth muscles in the walls of visceral organs and blood vessels also maintain tone or tension to prevent 'collapse' after emptying.

There are two types of smooth muscle: single-unit (unitary) and multi-unit. The two differ in location and characteristics. The unitary type has electrical synapses or gap junctions, which are low-resistance pathways enabling the fast spread of action potentials and synchronous contraction of muscle as a single

unit. Single-unit smooth muscle possesses inherent pacemaker activity or slow waves, which set the rhythm or frequency of spontaneous contractions. If this pacemaker activity is disrupted in the bladder, it leads to 'overactive bladder' and incontinence.

Unitary smooth muscle type is found in the walls of all visceral organs, except the heart (which has cardiac muscle in its walls), which are stimulated by stretch during filling.

Multi-unit smooth muscle cells are not electrically coupled. As a result, contraction does not spread from one cell to the next. Instead, it is confined to the cell that was originally stimulated. Multi-unit smooth muscles are not stimulated by stretch but by neural stimulation by postganglionic sympathetic and parasympathetic fibres of the autonomic system (ANS), which regulate their function. Multi-unit smooth muscle fibres also respond to circulating hormones. This type of tissue is found around large blood vessels, in the respiratory airways, and in the eyes.

The E-C coupling in smooth muscle is different from that seen in the skeletal muscle (or cardiac muscle). Because smooth muscle cells do not contain troponin, cross-bridge formation is not regulated by the troponin-tropomyosin complex but instead by the regulatory protein *calmodulin*. The Ca^{2+}-calmodulin complex then activates an enzyme called *myosin* (light chain) kinase, which, in turn, phosphorylates the myosin heads. The heads can then attach to actin-binding sites and pull on the thin filaments. The arrangement of the thin filaments is such that it causes the entire muscle fibre to contract and bulge in the centre by a corkscrew motion, unlike the skeletal muscle.

As smooth muscle is not under voluntary control like the skeletal muscle, the axons of ANS neurons do not form the highly organised NMJs. Instead, there exists a number of neurotransmitter-filled bulges called *varicosities* as the axon traverses the smooth muscle. A *varicosity* releases neurotransmitters into the synaptic cleft (Figure 3.10).

Clinical Relevance

Myasthenia gravis is an autoimmune disease which causes progressive damage to the NMJ, chronic muscular weakness, and fatigue. Antibodies against the ACh receptors reduce the number of functional receptors at the motor end plate, impairing the action

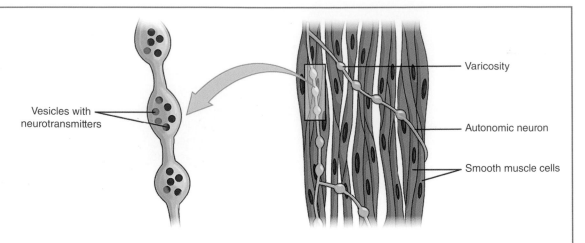

Figure 3.10 Motor units in smooth muscle. A series of axon-like swelling, called *varicosities* or boutons, from autonomic neurons form motor units throughout the smooth muscle. *Source:* OpenStax (2013).

of ACh and result in muscle weakness and fatigue. It occurs in 1 in 10 000 people, and initially muscles of the face and neck are often the first to be affected. The weakness of eye muscles can cause double vision followed by difficulty in swallowing, chewing, and speech as the disease progresses. If left untreated, the disease may paralyse limb and respiratory muscles.

Tetany is a state of sustained involuntary contraction of muscles (Chapter 19). This happens if a muscle is repeatedly stimulated, causing accumulation of high levels of Ca^{2+} in the sarcoplasm (due to insufficient time for Ca^{2+} to move the ions back into sarcoplasmic reticulum). The elevated Ca^{2+} results in continued binding of the ion to troponin C and cross-bridge formation, leading to sustained contraction called *tetany*, rather than just a single twitch.

Cranial nerve neuropathies may result from nerve damage and lead to impaired motor and/or sensory function (Chapter 21).

Botulinum toxin reduces the release of ACh at the nerve terminals and blocks neuromuscular transmission, leading to flaccid muscular paralysis. It has several clinical applications, including the treatment of the *strabismus* (crossed eyes), *spasms of vocal cords*, *blepharospasm* (uncontrollable blinking), and overactive bladder. Botulinum toxin is also used for the cosmetic treatment of facial wrinkles and acts by impairing the contraction of facial muscles.

Hypertrophy of the masseter muscles may be caused by tooth grinding habits (Bruxism) resulting in facial asymmetry and/or a squarish appearance of

the face (Chapter 9). Gross masseteric hypertrophy may be treated by botulinum toxin.

References

OpenStax (2013). Smooth muscle. In: Anatomy and Physiology. Rice University created under Creative Commons Attribution 4.0 International License, OpenStax, Montreal, Canada https://opentextbc.ca/anatomyandphysiology/chapter/10-8-smooth-muscle (accessed 1 May 2018).

Tortora, G.J. and Derrickson, B. (2017). The muscular tissue. In: *Principles of Anatomy and Physiology*, 15e, 293–329. Wiley.

Further Reading

Hasudungan, A. (2012a). Skeletal muscle (sarcomere, myosin and actin). https://www.youtube.com/watch?v=MZJ6kTKDFmw (accessed 3 May 2018).

Hasudungan, A. (2012b). Skeletal muscle contraction. https://www.youtube.com/watch?v=Vs0tZV35_pw (accessed 3 May 2018).

Mc-Graw Hill Animations (2017). Muscle contraction process. https://www.youtube.com/watch?v=ousflrOzQHc (accessed 3 May 2018).

Sherwood, L. (2016). Muscle physiology. In: *Human Physiology: From Cells to System*, 9e, 251–296. Boston: Cengage Learning.

Silverthorn, D.U. (2017). Muscle. In: *Human Physiology: An Integrated Approach*, 7e, 401–440. Pearson Education.

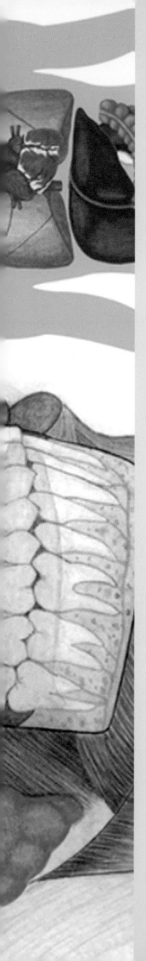

PART III
Cardiovascular System

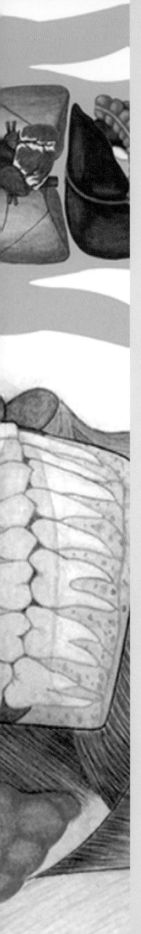

CHAPTER 4
Heart

Poorna Gunasekera, Kamran Ali, and Elizabeth Prabhakar

Key Topics

- Overview of the structure and functions of the heart
- Common cardiac diseases

Learning Objectives

To demonstrate an understanding of the:

- Gross anatomy, histology and properties of the heart
- Organisation of the pulmonary and systemic circulation
- Conduction system of the heart and the cardiac cycle
- Common cardiac indices
- Common disorders of the heart and their relevance to the provision of dental care

Introduction

The human heart measures approximately the size of a clenched fist and could be described as a 'toppled pyramid' resting on its side, with the apex placed inferiorly and pointing towards the left anterior surface and the base pointing posteriorly to the right. This results in almost two-thirds of the heart lying on the left of the midline, with the right ventricle occupying a major part of the anterior surface deep to the chest wall. The heart is located in the mid-thoracic space between the two lungs (mediastinum) with the great vessels (the aorta and the pulmonary trunk) exiting the base.

Gross Anatomy

The heart is essentially a hollow cavity surrounded by a fibromuscular wall and is divided into four chambers separated by valves and septa. This wall has three layers, from superficial to deep: *pericardium*, *myocardium*, and *endocardium* (Figure 4.1).

Essential Physiology for Dental Students, First Edition. Edited by Kamran Ali and Elizabeth Prabhakar.
© 2019 John Wiley & Sons Ltd. Published 2019 by John Wiley & Sons Ltd.
Companion website: www.wiley.com/go/ali/physiology

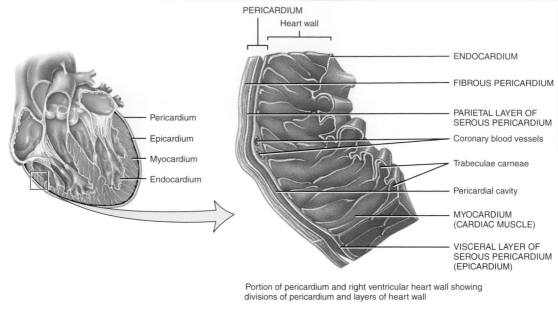

PERICARDIUM

Heart wall

ENDOCARDIUM

FIBROUS PERICARDIUM

PARIETAL LAYER OF SEROUS PERICARDIUM

Coronary blood vessels

Trabeculae carneae

Pericardial cavity

MYOCARDIUM (CARDIAC MUSCLE)

VISCERAL LAYER OF SEROUS PERICARDIUM (EPICARDIUM)

Pericardium

Epicardium

Myocardium

Endocardium

Portion of pericardium and right ventricular heart wall showing divisions of pericardium and layers of heart wall

Figure 4.1 Layers of the heart wall. *Source:* Tortora and Derrickson (2013).

The pericardium is composed of two layers: the outer tough fibrous pericardium and the inner serous pericardium. The fibrous pericardium is continuous with the tunica adventitia of the great vessels superiorly and fuses with the diaphragm inferiorly. The serous pericardium is itself made of two layers: the outer parietal pericardium and the inner visceral pericardium. The space between these two layers is filled by pericardial fluid. The visceral pericardium is also called the epicardium.

The middle myocardium is by far the thickest layer and is almost entirely composed of the parenchymatous tissue of the heart: the cardiomyocytes (cardiocytes). The innermost endocardium is made of a single layer of cells that is continuous with the endothelium of the blood vessels entering or exiting the heart.

Cardiac Chambers

The heart could be described as two individual pumps (right and left) that are located next to each other. The four chambers of the heart consist of two atria (upper chambers) and two ventricles (lower chambers). The atria have thinner fibromuscular walls than the ventricles, because blood is only pumped a short distance (atria to ventricles). The left ventricle has the thickest myocardium compared to the other three chambers, because it has to generate a forceful contraction (to maintain high pressure) in order to pump blood the great distances in the body.

The right side of the body carries deoxygenated blood, while the left side of the body carries oxygenated blood. The left and right atria are separated by the interatrial septum. The interventricular septum separates the left and right ventricles, ensuring that deoxygenated blood and oxygenated blood do not mix.

Cardiac Valves

The atria and ventricles are connected to each other by openings that contain valves to facilitate one-way flow. These are known as atrioventricular (AV) valves (Figure 4.2). The valve between the right atrium and right ventricle is known as the tricuspid valve, and has three cusps as the name implies. The valve between the left atrium and left ventricle is the only one to have two cusps, and is known as the *mitral* or *bicuspid valve.*

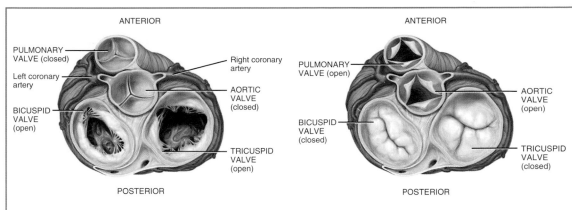

Figure 4.2 Cardiac valves. *Source:* Tortora and Derrickson (2013).

Similarly, the points of exit of the great vessels from the ventricles also contain valves, which are named after the great vessels themselves (i.e. the aortic and the pulmonary valves). Both valves have three cusps each.

As the AV valves must resist the pressures caused by ventricular contraction, they contain a series of tough fibrous cord-like tendons, known as *chordae tendineae* (or commonly referred to as heart strings), which anchor the margin of the cusps to the underside of their ventricular surfaces, and prevent inversion backwards into the atria. The chordae tendineae are in turn attached to the ventricular wall by papillary muscles, which contract during systole (ventricular contraction), thereby tensing the chordae tendineae and therefore the valves. Some chordae tendineae may arise directly from the myocardium or the interventricular septum.

Neurovascular Supply

The heart receives postganglionic sympathetic supply from the sympathetic chain which innervates most of the cardiac tissues. The postganglionic parasympathetic nerves originate from the cardiac plexus, which is located very close to the pericardium. This parasympathetic innervation is mostly to the two main centres that are responsible for maintaining the cardiac rhythm: the sinoatrial (SA) and the AV nodes.

The myocardium is perfused by two coronary arteries (right and left) that branch from the origin of the aorta. The venous blood from most of the coronary circulation collects into the great vein, which drains into the right atrium through the coronary sinus.

The lymphatic drainage returns excessive interstitial fluid or lymph into venous circulation from the right and left sides of the body via lymph trunks, which drain into jugulars and subclavian veins. The lymph eventually drains into the superior vena cava via the right and left brachiocephalic veins.

Pulmonary and Systemic Circulation

The right atrium receives venous (deoxygenated) blood via the superior and inferior *venae cavae* (from the head and rest of body, respectively, excluding lungs). It also receives blood from the coronary sinus, which carries venous blood from the epicardial circulation (the blood supply to the heart muscle itself). The right ventricle pumps out blood into the pulmonary trunk, which divides into the right and left pulmonary arteries, which transport deoxygenated blood to the respective lungs for oxygenation.

The oxygenated blood from the lungs is returned to the left atrium via four pulmonary veins, through pulmonary circulation. The left atrium then pumps blood into the left ventricle and then into the systemic circulation via the aorta (Figure 4.3). The separation of heart circulation into two divisions: systemic and pulmonary is called *double circulation*.

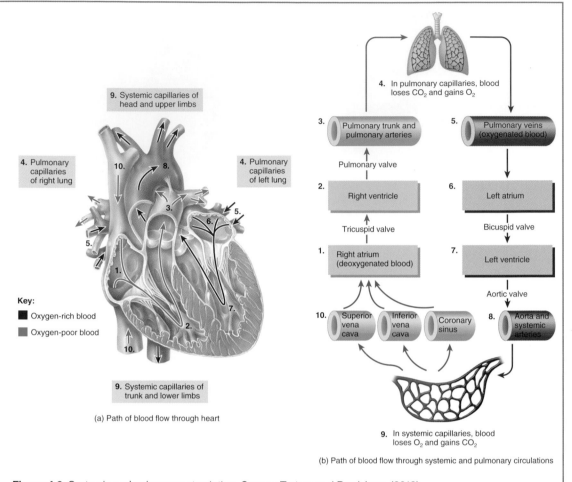

9. Systemic capillaries of head and upper limbs

4. Pulmonary capillaries of right lung

10.

8.

3.

5.

6.

4. Pulmonary capillaries of left lung

5.

1.

7.

2.

10.

Key:
■ Oxygen-rich blood
■ Oxygen-poor blood

9. Systemic capillaries of trunk and lower limbs

(a) Path of blood flow through heart

4. In pulmonary capillaries, blood loses CO_2 and gains O_2

3. Pulmonary trunk and pulmonary arteries

5. Pulmonary veins (oxygenated blood)

Pulmonary valve

2. Right ventricle

6. Left atrium

Tricuspid valve

Bicuspid valve

1. Right atrium (deoxygenated blood)

7. Left ventricle

Aortic valve

10. Superior vena cava | Inferior vena cava | Coronary sinus

8. Aorta and systemic arteries

9. In systemic capillaries, blood loses O_2 and gains CO_2

(b) Path of blood flow through systemic and pulmonary circulations

Figure 4.3 Systemic and pulmonary circulation. *Source:* Tortora and Derrickson (2013).

Functional Histology

The Functional Cell: Cardiocyte

The myocardium is almost exclusively made up of cardiocytes which are classified as involuntary muscle. The cardiac muscle (Figure 4.4) is striated like the skeletal muscle (Chapter 3). However, certain features of the cardiac muscle are quite distinct and discussed below.

A typical cardiocyte has a single central nucleus and is connected to many other cells through intercalated discs (Figure 4.4). The intercalated discs have a step-shaped configuration with longitudinal and transverse components that are continuous with one another. The irregular transverse components are thickenings of the sarcolemma, which are placed at right angles to the long axes of the cells and contain desmosomes and connect one cardiac muscle cell to another. The longitudinal components, which run parallel to the length of the cardiocyte, contain *gap junctions* (electrical synapses), which enable rapid ionic communication between adjoining cells, causing contraction of the cardiac muscle as a coordinated single unit. This function is facilitated by the movement of calcium, which is essential in triggering the depolarisation. The cardiac action potential uniquely causes a contraction which lasts about 15 times longer than the contraction of the skeletal muscle, owing to the sustained release of calcium, and its long refractory period which prevents fatigue.

The cardiocytes contain numerous mitochondria providing an abundant supply of energy to facilitate rhythmic muscle contraction. The contraction is

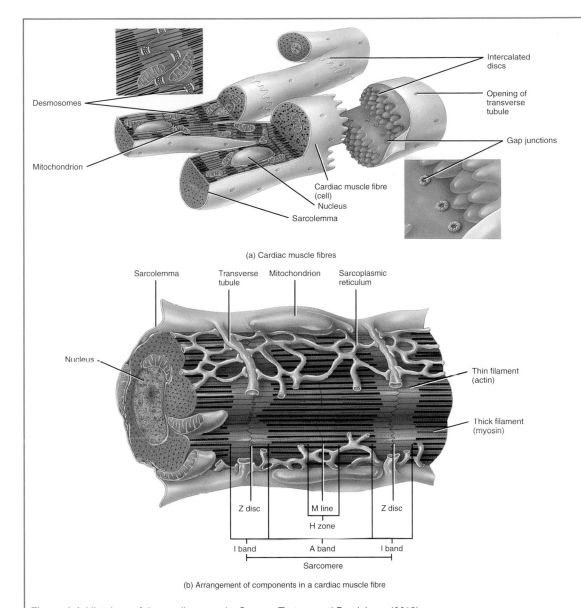

(a) Cardiac muscle fibres

(b) Arrangement of components in a cardiac muscle fibre

Figure 4.4 Histology of the cardiac muscle. *Source:* Tortora and Derrickson (2013).

brought about by the overlap of actin and myosin myofilaments on each other, which is very similar to the mechanism seen in skeletal muscle contraction.

Conduction System

The conduction system originates in the SA node, which is found close to the entry point of the superior *venae cavae* into the right atrium (Figure 4.5).

From here, the electrical impulses (action potentials) travel down inter-nodal pathways to the AV node, which is situated in the lowest part of the interatrial septum. The impulses are then carried through the interventricular septum by the Atrioventricular bundle, also known as the *bundle of His*, which is made of a single right branch and two left branches. These branches then divide into a series of Purkinje fibres which travel upwards on all sides from the apex of the

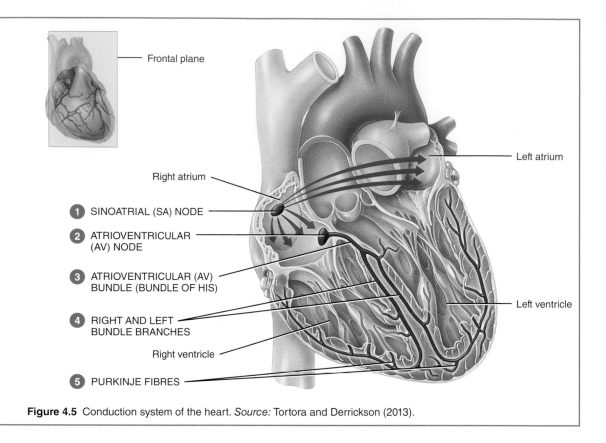

Frontal plane

Left atrium

Right atrium

1 SINOATRIAL (SA) NODE

2 ATRIOVENTRICULAR (AV) NODE

3 ATRIOVENTRICULAR (AV) BUNDLE (BUNDLE OF HIS)

4 RIGHT AND LEFT BUNDLE BRANCHES

Left ventricle

Right ventricle

5 PURKINJE FIBRES

Figure 4.5 Conduction system of the heart. *Source:* Tortora and Derrickson (2013).

heart, very much like the spokes of an umbrella. The electrical impulses can only travel from the atria to the ventricles through the AV node. The cardiac skeleton, which provides the frame for the four cardiac valves, prevents the passage of impulses through any other locations.

Cardiac Contractility

SA Node Autorhythmicity or Pacemaker Activity

Though the heart muscle is innervated by the autonomic nervous system (ANS), it does not rely on nerve stimulation to initiate impulses. This is because approximately 1% of cardiocytes (autorhythmic fibres or pacemaker cells) found in the SA node (Figure 4.5) are inherently self-excitable or myogenic, unlike the skeletal muscle, which is neurogenic. A denervated heart will continue to beat, as happens during a transplant procedure. Thus, the pacemaker cells set the rhythm of the

heart to a rapid 100 beats per minute (bpm), which is normally decreased to an average of 72 bpm, by the release of acetylcholine from postganglionic parasympathetic nerves.

Pacemaker cells are able to generate impulses spontaneously because they have unstable or drifting resting potentials (pacemaker potentials), owing to sodium leakage through '*funny channels*' in the cell membrane. The influx of sodium through *funny channels* depolarises the cell towards a threshold of –40 mV. At threshold, fast voltage-gated calcium channels open and allow calcium into the cells to elicit *pacemaker action potentials* (Figure 4.6).

These action potentials are transmitted along conduction pathways in the heart. When the wave of excitation reaches the *contractile cells* (the 'working' cells) located in the chambers of the heart, they are depolarised to produce *contractile action potentials*, which have shapes distinctive to those of pacemaker action potentials. A contractile action potential has three phases which are dependent on

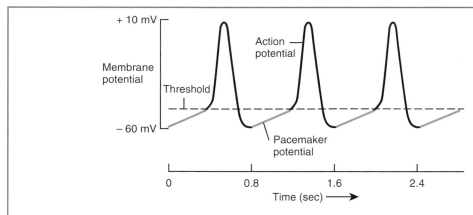

Figure 4.6 Pacemaker potentials (green) and action potentials (black) in autorhythmic fibres of SA node. *Source:* Tortora and Derrickson (2013).

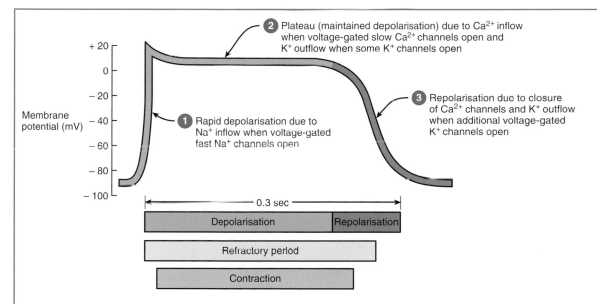

Figure 4.7 Action potentials in ventricular contractile fibre (resting membrane potential –90 mV). *Source:* Tortora and Derrickson (2013).

the opening and closing of voltage-gated ion channels in the sarcolemma: Phase 1, upstroke of action potential or depolarisation due to sodium influx; Phase 2, 'plateau' phase or sustained depolarisation caused by calcium influx, which stimulates the release of more calcium the sarcoplasmic reticulum; and, finally; Phase 3, repolarisation due to potassium efflux (Figure 4.7). The contractile action potentials initiate systolic and diastolic events in the cardiac cycle.

Cardiac Cycle

The rhythmic pumping of the heart enabled by the 'cardiac cycle', facilitates blood flow through the vessels of the systemic and pulmonary circulatory systems. The main events associated with the cardiac cycle are atrial systole, ventricular systole and diastole, described below (Figure 4.8).

The cardiac cycle, which is initiated by the pacemaker activity, results in action potentials which can be recorded as an electrocardiogram (ECG). The ECG has characteristic waves: the *P-wave* (Figure 4.8a, point 1), which triggers the contraction of atria in a 'domino-like' fashion, to propel blood contained within the atria towards the open atrio-ventricular orifice. This event is named *atrial systole* (Figure 4.8b, point 2), which marks the final emptying of the blood from the atria to the

ventricles (called "*atrial kick*"), which occurs in the phase referred to as diastole. Please note therefore, that atrial systole occurs during 'normal' diastole. The impulses that originate from the SA node travel down to the AV node using two routes (i) fast internodal path and (ii) the slower passage via surface membranes of contracting atrial cardiocytes.

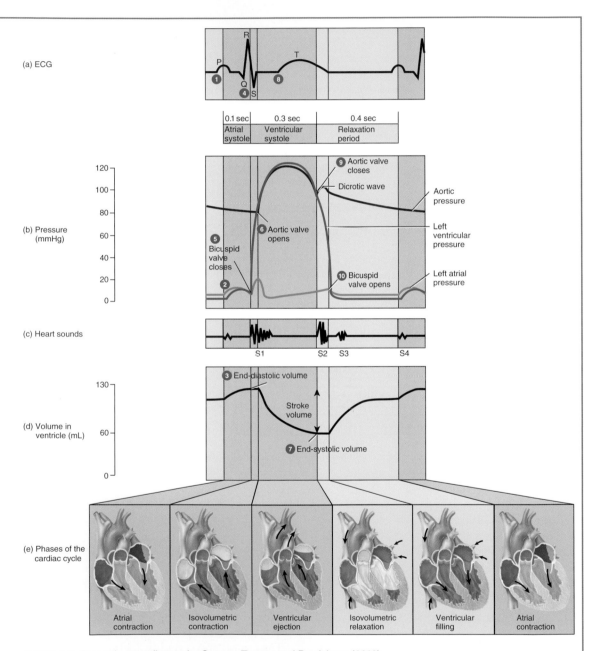

Figure 4.8 Events in a cardiac cycle. *Source:* Tortora and Derrickson (2013).

At the AV node, there is a pause (dubbed AV nodal delay) in impulse conduction of 100–120 ms or 0.12 s, which is vital for the atria to complete their contraction. The blood that pools in each ventricle at the end of atrial systole is known as the end-diastolic volume (Figure 4.8d, point 3). The AV node now 'releases' the impulses, which travel rapidly down the Bundle of His towards the apex of the heart to fan out in all directions, towards the base via Purkinje fibres, to depolarise ventricles. This event is marked by the QRS complex on ECG (Figure 4.8a, point 4), which leads to ventricular systole or the contraction of ventricles.

The contracting ventricles force the blood towards the base, making the cusps of the AV valves to move upwards till their margins come to oppose one another. Further contraction forces the valve cusps to shut and prevent backflow of blood to the atria (Figure 4.8b, point 5). Valve closure also produces the first 'lub' heart sound (S1) as shown in Figure 4.8c. In this, systolic phase, the ventricular pressure continues to rise (owing to the contraction of the chamber wall) without producing a concomitant change in blood volume, called *isovolumetric contraction* (Figure 4.8e).

The ventricles continue to contract even after the AV valves close, which further increases ventricular pressure until it overcomes the pressures within the great vessels (i.e. aorta and pulmonary trunk). When the pressures within each chamber exceed those within the vessels, they force open the semilunar valves (aortic and pulmonary valves), thereby facilitating the passage of blood from the ventricles into the great vessels (Figure 4.8b, point 6). This results in the 'emptying' of the chamber, though in most instances some residual blood remains within each ventricle. The heart continues to contract throughout this period, where each ventricle empties into the corresponding great vessel without a marked change of the pressures in each chamber.

The contraction of the cardiac muscles ceases with the completion of the passage of each action potential over their surface membrane. The period of relaxation that follows leads to a rapid drop in the pressure within each chamber. The moment the pressure within each chamber drops below the pressures within their respective great vessels, there is a tendency for the blood within the vessels to flow back towards the chamber it was just pumped out from. This back flow is prevented by the shutting of the semilunar valves, i.e. aortic and pulmonary or pulmonic valves (Figure 4.8b, point 9). Closure of the semi-lunar valves produces the second heart sound known as 'dub' (S2) as shown in Figure 4.8c. This marks the end of systole. The volume of blood remaining in each chamber at this point is known as the *end-systolic volume* ((Figure 4.8d, point 7). The repolarisation of the ventricles, in preparation for the next wave of depolarisation, is marked by the T wave of the ECG (Figure 4.8a, point 8).

Despite the heart no longer 'pumping blood' actively, the blood flow continues in the venous compartment helped by forces such as the contraction of surrounding tissues, especially muscles. Moreover, the negative thoracic pressure caused by inspiration also helps 'suck' blood back towards the atria. This results in a passive filling of the heart: the period of diastole.

The continued drop in ventricular pressures during diastole will lead to a point where the pressures are below those in the respective atria. This period where the pressure within the ventricles continues to drop without any change in the volume of blood contained within them is called isovolumetric relaxation. (Figure 4.8e)

The moment intraventricular pressures drop below that within the atria, the AV valves are pushed open towards the ventricles (Figure 4.8e, point 10), thereby ushering the filling of the ventricles, without any change in pressure (as the ventricles expand passively), the period of isotonic relaxation. This period is ended by the new initiation of an impulse from the SA node, leading to a new wave of atrial contraction, the atrial diastole.

Cardiac Indices

The various phases of cardiac contraction give rise to indices that are vital in assessing the health status of individuals. For instance, the period between two cardiac contractions (i.e. one cycle of systole followed by diastole) is known as a *cardiac cycle*. The total number of cardiac cycles per minute is known as the heart rate. The volume of blood pumped out from one ventricle (conventionally the left) during one systole is known as the *stroke volume* (SV). The total amount of blood pumped from one ventricle (conventionally the left) per minute is known as the *cardiac output* (CO).

This leads to the equation: CO = HR × SV. While there could be individual variation, as for instance seen in professional athletes, the heart rate of a healthy adult ranges generally between 60 and 100 bpm. The stroke volume may range from 60 to 100 ml per minute. This translates into a cardiac output of between 4 and 8 l^{-1}.

Various other indices, such as ejection fraction of each ventricle (the volume of blood pumped out during systole as a fraction of the volume of blood that filled the chamber at the end of diastole), are also used when evaluating cardiac function.

Other Functions

In addition to the main function of pumping blood, the heart also contributes to the endocrine system. It does so through specialised cells that secrete atrial natriuretic peptide (ANP) from the right atrium and brain natriuretic peptide (BNP) from the ventricles. Both ANP and BNP function as natural opponents to the actions of angiotensin II (Chapter 17).

Clinical Relevance

Ischaemic heart disease (IHD) is a group of conditions which results from a reduction in coronary blood flow and is the commonest type of cardiac disease. IHD presents with acute chest pain which may radiate to the shoulder, back, neck, and the lower jaw. Patients with IHD are often prescribed blood thinners to reduce the risk of cardiac events which increase the risk of bleeding during dental surgical procedures (Chapter 16). Stress and anxiety associated with dental treatment may precipitate acute chest pain in patients with a history of IHD and constitute a medical emergency.

Cardiac arrest is a potentially fatal condition characterised by loss of consciousness due to sudden cessation of cardiac function. It may result from cardiac or respiratory causes. Dental professionals need training in basic life support (BLS) for the management of cardiac arrest in line with the national guidelines.

Patients with prosthetic heart valves and certain types of congenital heart disease are at risk of bacterial *endocarditis* (infection of the endocardium) due to bacteraemia from the oral cavity. Dental professionals need to evaluate the need for prophylactic antibiotics in patients at risk of endocarditis by liaising with medical colleagues.

Sudden death: genetic diseases caused by abnormally shaped voltage-gated ion channels can result in abnormal heart rhythms, like atrial fibrillation, tachycardia or bradycardia. Undiagnosed conditions could lead to cardiac arrest or sudden death syndrome.

Reference

Tortora, G.J. and Derrickson, B. (2013). *Principles of Anatomy and Physiology*. Hoboken, NJ: Wiley.

Further Reading

Campbell, J. (2018). Cardiovascular system 1: Heart, structure and function. https://www.youtube.com/watch?v=VWamhZ8vTL4 (accessed 1 May 2018).

Courses Washington Edu (2018). Cardiac action potentials. https://courses.washington.edu/conj/heart/cardiacAP2011.htm (accessed 1 May 2018).

Dr Najeeb Lectures (2018). Cardiac cycle: Systole & diastole: Part 1/8. https://www.youtube.com/watch?v=XbivIaFPoQI&list=PL012959432554AE8E (accessed 1 May 2018).

Pinnell, J., Turner, S., and Howell, S. (2007). Cardiac muscle physiology. *Continuing Education in Anaesthesia Critical Care & Pain* 7 (3): 85–88.

Sherwood, L. (2016). Cardiac physiology. In: *Human Physiology: From Cells to Systems*, vol. 9, 297–334. Boston: Cengage Learning.

Tortora, G.J. and Derrickson, B. (2017). The cardiovascular system. In: *Principles of Anatomy and Physiology*, 695–736. Hoboken, NJ: Wiley.

CHAPTER 5
Circulation

Poorna Gunasekera and Kamran Ali

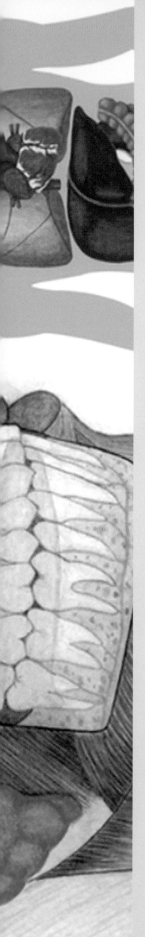

Key Topics

- Overview of circulatory system
- Common disorders of the circulatory system

Learning Objectives

To demonstrate an understanding of the:

- Functional organisation of the circulatory system
- Types and functions of blood vessels
- Regulation of circulation and blood pressure
- Common disorders of blood circulation and their impact on provision of dental care

Introduction

The circulatory system is made up of a series of interconnecting tubes (blood vessels) that carry blood to and from the heart. Together with the heart, these form the *cardio-vascular system*, which plays a vital role in transporting nutrients to the cells, carrying away cellular waste products to excretory organs such as the kidneys, the lungs, and the liver. In addition, the circulatory system contributes to the efficient functioning of the immune system by providing a mode for cells and cellular products (such as immunoglobulins) to move quickly throughout the body. Similarly, it provides an essential supporting function for the endocrine system by transporting hormones. It further contributes to homeostasis by helping to maintain the *interior milieu* via the pH buffering action of haemoglobin in the blood and the maintenance of body temperature.

The different components of the circulatory system serve specialised functions and are named accordingly. By far the largest of such arrangements, the *systemic circulation*

Essential Physiology for Dental Students, First Edition. Edited by Kamran Ali and Elizabeth Prabhakar.
© 2019 John Wiley & Sons Ltd. Published 2019 by John Wiley & Sons Ltd.
Companion website: www.wiley.com/go/ali/physiology

(Chapter 4), accounts for the transport of blood from the left ventricle to all major organs of the body (except the lungs) and its return to the right atrium. The *pulmonary system*, in comparison, is much smaller and facilitates the movement of blood from the right ventricle to the lungs and its return to the left atrium. The *entero-hepatic system* is another important arrangement whereby venous-blood-carrying nutrients absorbed from the gastro-intestinal (GIT) system are carried to the liver, before draining into the systemic circulation via the hepatic veins.

Classification

The vessels that form the circulatory system are categorised as *arteries*, *veins*, and *capillaries*. The arteries are defined as vessels that carry blood away from the heart, while veins are vessels that carry blood towards the heart. These two systems of tubes are connected peripherally through capillaries. Owing to this nomenclature, the blood vessels that carry blood away from the heart to the lungs are classified as *pulmonary arteries*, even though they carry deoxygenated blood. Correspondingly, pulmonary veins return oxygenated blood to the heart. This is repeated in foetal circulation, where a single umbilical vein carries relatively more oxygenated blood towards the foetal heart, while two umbilical arteries carry deoxygenated blood towards the placenta, away from the foetal heart.

The blood vessels vary in calibre as well as thickness. They can be described as having multi-layered walls which progressively reduce in thickness as they move away from the heart towards the interconnecting capillaries, which have the thinnest walls. This arrangement is vital to the progressive increase in blood volume found within vessels in close proximity to the heart, as well as to facilitate the exchange of soluble components between the fluid contained in the vascular compartment and fluid found in tissue spaces (interstitial fluid) in the peripheries.

The arteries therefore branch repeatedly distributing blood through progressively smaller calibre (diameter), forming greater numbers of arterioles (forming the arterial tree) as they carry blood away from the heart towards the capillaries. The venules drain blood from these capillaries and coalesce to form larger veins, thereby collecting progressively greater volumes of blood as they move towards the heart. In systemic circulation, this arrangement is

completed by a single aorta that leaves the left ventricle of the heart, and two great veins, the superior and inferior *venae cavae*, which drain the blood back to the right atrium. A network of capillaries join the arterioles of the aorta and venules of the venae cavae.

Functional Histology

All blood vessels, regardless of their calibre and thickness, are lined on their internal surfaces by a single layer of squamous cells, collectively called the *endothelium*, which is continuous with the endocardium lining the innermost surface of the heart wall. Because this layer is in immediate contact with the blood contained within the lumen of the vessels, it is known as the *tunic interna* (and sometimes the *tunica intima*). A basement membrane made up of acellular material lies immediately on the external surface of the endothelial cells, providing mechanical support for the tunica intima. The capillary walls are made up of only these two layers: the singular layer of endothelial cells and surrounding basement membrane (Figure 5.1).

Arteries and veins, in contrast, have further layers of tissue contributing to their walls. A second layer of tissue, comprising smooth muscle cells, surrounds the tunica intima and is termed the *tunica media*. The layer of acellular material that lies between the cells of the tunica intima and media is called the *internal elastic lamina*. The tunica media, in turn, has an outermost layer of tissue that helps attach the blood vessels to surrounding tissue such as skeletal muscle. This layer is called the *tunica externa* (also known as the *tunica adventitia*), with another layer of acellular material, the *external elastic lamina*, lying between it and the inner tunica media.

The thickness of blood vessel walls is largely determined by the multiplicity of the smooth muscles cells in the tunica media. As a rule, arteries have more smooth muscles than veins. This arrangement enables arteries to accommodate the pressure of blood that is forcefully pumped out from the heart during systole, by the active relaxation of smooth muscle. The veins, in contrast, by having a relatively thinner wall, are able to expand to provide a space for a greater volume of blood to be stored within their lumen when it is not needed, a quality which is recognised in the term *capacitance vessels*. The arteries are accordingly called *resistance vessels* as they resist the pressure of blood pumped out from

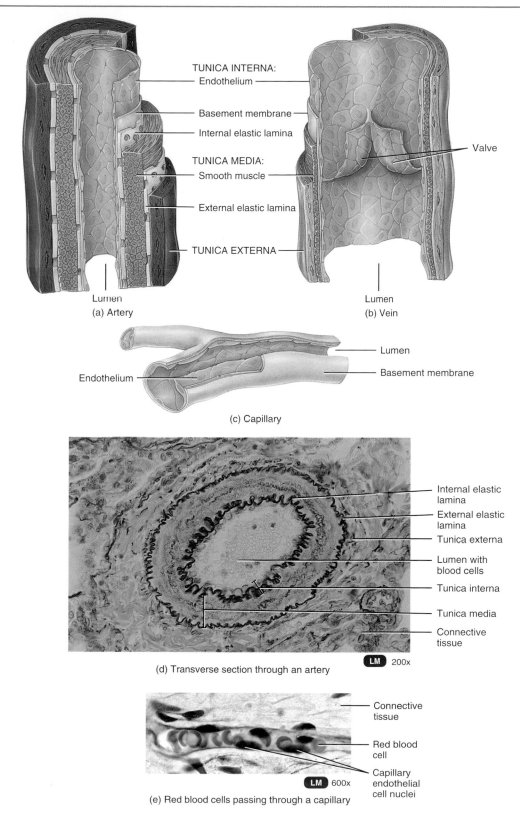

Figure 5.1 Comparative structure of blood vessels. *Source:* Tortora and Derrickson (2013).

the heart. One other functional adaptation in veins is that they have valves in their internal lumen; this prevents the backflow of blood during its return to the heart from the periphery.

Determinants of Circulation

This arrangement of arteries carrying blood away from the heart and veins returning that blood, with the two tubular systems connected at the periphery through capillaries, enables the continuous one-way flow of blood and is termed *circulation*. There are several important factors at play to facilitate uninterrupted, continuous circulation and to prevent stagnation at any point.

Rhythmic Contraction of the Heart

The force for the propulsion of blood through the *arterial tree* (the complex of major arteries dividing into progressively smaller and more numerous smaller arteries and arterioles, which ultimately lead to capillaries) is provided by the rhythmic contraction of the heart during ventricular systole. The smooth muscles within arterial walls actively relax immediately prior to the outflow of blood ejected during systole, thereby distending the lumen within the vessels, which serves to reduce the resistance the heart would otherwise have to overcome.

Soon after the initial bolus of the ejected blood volume passes a particular point in an artery, there is a release of the elastic energy generated during the process of active distension, leading to a contraction of the arterial walls. This sequence of distension followed by contraction facilitates the continuous flow of blood. This is achieved by accommodating the rapid increase of blood volume during systole, and then contracting to sustain sufficient pressure to maintain the velocity of blood flow during diastole, when blood is no longer being pumped by the heart. These changes are reflected in the systolic and diastolic arterial blood pressure readings that are widely used indices in measuring cardiovascular health. This 'pulse wave' of distension followed by contraction of the arteries travels down the length of the arterial tree, originating from the root of the aorta, and facilitates the rapid flow of blood towards the periphery.

While the events associated with the pulse wave may provide sufficient force to propel blood from the heart to the peripheral capillaries, it then faces the challenge of finding means to return to the heart to maintain continuous circulation. As there is no 'peripheral heart' to propel blood actively from the capillaries to the heart, its return journey is facilitated by passive forces that affect the venous compartment. These include the contraction of relatively thin walled venous vessels by adjacent structures. Notably, the soleus muscle, found in the calf region, plays an invaluable role in contracting the veins within it, especially when moving about in an upright posture, a property acknowledged by the term *skeletal-muscle pump*. While the compression of the walls of the veins, owing to forces such as muscle contraction, helps displace the blood within their lumens, the valves ensure the displacement only occurs in one direction, thereby facilitating the one-way flow of blood.

Another factor that contributes to the return of venous blood is the negative intrathoracic pressure caused by the expansion of the rib cage during inspiration. This literally helps suck the blood away from the peripheries, such as the abdomen, back towards the lumen of the right atrium. It is important to note that the heart itself does not actively contribute to the return of venous blood; venous blood fills relaxing cardiac chambers during diastole.

Determinants of Arterial Blood Pressure

While arterial blood pressure is a key determinant of cardiovascular health, its increase beyond safe limits is the defining feature of hypertension. In the study of haemodynamics (the mechanisms of blood flow), two factors are recognised as the main contributors to blood pressure (BP) in general. One is cardiac output (CO), which is a measure of the blood volume pumped from one ventricle (conventionally the left) in one minute and the other is *total peripheral resistance* (TPR, also known as *systemic vascular resistance*, or SVR), which is a measure of the resistance offered by the arterial tree that the heart must overcome to expel blood during systole. The relationship between these variables is shown in the equation $BP = CO \times TPR$.

While this is not a mathematical equation, it identifies the key variables that can be altered when attempting to maintain BP within healthy limits. As CO is a direct measure of the stroke volume (SV) multiplied by heart rate (HR – beats per minute), this demonstrates that reductions in TPR (which is largely determined by resistance in the arterioles), SV, or HR are all effective in reducing the overall BP.

A multitude of feedback mechanisms plays a vital role in maintaining BP within physiological limits. For instance, when a person stands up from a recumbent position, this leads to a rapid pooling of blood in the lower extremities, owing to gravitational forces. This results in a momentary fall in the volume of blood in the rest of the circulatory system, leading to a drop in BP. This is detected by pressure receptors (baroreceptors) in the carotid sinuses and the arch of the aorta, afferent nerves which relay this information to the cardiac centre in the medulla oblongata. This in turn leads to a reflex increase of the sympathetic outflow to the heart and a reduction of the parasympathetic stimulation. This, together with increased secretion of adrenaline and noradrenaline from the adrenal medulla, results in an increase in HR as well as the SV, coupled with an increase of TPR, all of which contributes to restoring the BP to its 'normal' value (Figure 5.2).

This same feedback system is also responsible for maintaining BP, and therefore circulation, in pathological states such as hypovolaemic shock resulting from sudden and excessive loss of blood (Figure 5.3).

Variations in Regional Blood Flow

While the mechanisms described above help in maintaining the flow of blood to and from the heart continuously, not all blood vessels are filled with blood throughout each cycle. At least in the mesenteric circulation (the network that perfuses the small and large intestines and transports absorbed nutrients), the smallest arterioles from which capillary networks branch off (sometimes referred to as *metarterioles*) are equipped with a discontinuous layer of smooth muscle cells, forming 'pre-capillary sphincters'. These sphincters can effectively limit the flow of blood into the capillary network (the capillary bed) based on the need for local perfusion. The sphincters may therefore contract to keep a limited number of capillaries open (called *thoroughfare channels*) when the tissue is in a resting state, but relax to flood the capillary bed with blood at times of greater activity, as would manifest soon after a meal when the ingested food

has to be digested and absorbed within a limited period of time.

Coagulation and Fibrinolytic Systems

The sheer stress caused by the rapid and continuous flow of blood within the lumen and other external forces may damage the walls of blood vessels, increasing the possibility of leaks. This is countered by a *coagulation system*, formed of platelets and soluble precursors called *coagulation factors*, which can rapidly be stimulated to sequentially form insoluble *fibrin* strands that manifest as clots within the vessels.

As much as such clots (known as *thrombi*) may prevent the leakage of blood from damaged vessels, they can also potentially occlude the blood vessels, blocking the flow of blood to the organs that rely on them for perfusion. This is averted by a *fibrinolytic system*, which breaks down the insoluble fibrin strands to ensure the clot does not persist for any longer than is necessary.

Fluid Compartments of the Body

Approximately 55–60% of the bodyweight of a human is made up of fluid, which is contained within three 'compartments' of the body. By far the largest collection, amounting to about 60% of the total body fluid, is found within cells, which is thus known as the *intracellular compartment*. Fluid found outside cells is thus known as *extracellular fluid*.

The second-largest fluid compartment, the interstitial space, is found immediately outside the cells, forming an ill-defined, fluid-filled layer between the fluid contained within cells and that found within the blood vessels of the circulatory system. Correspondingly, fluid found within the lumen of the blood vessels is called the *intravascular fluid*, thus making all fluid outside the lumen (i.e. the intracellular and interstitial fluid) to be known collectively as *extravascular fluid*. In a normal human, intravascular fluid accounts for approximately 10% of total body fluid, while the remaining 30% is found within the interstitial space. The intravascular fluid, together with the cellular elements contained within the lumen of the vessels of the circulatory system, is collectively called *blood*.

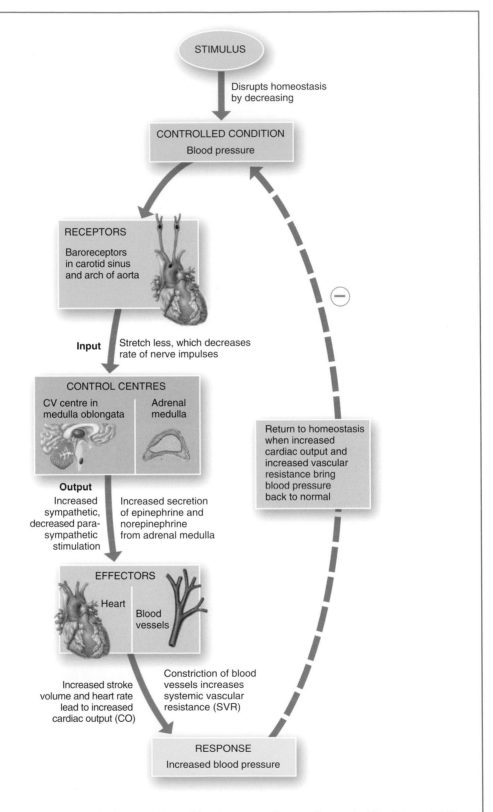

Figure 5.2 Role of baroreceptors in the regulation of blood pressure. *Source:* Tortora and Derrickson (2013).

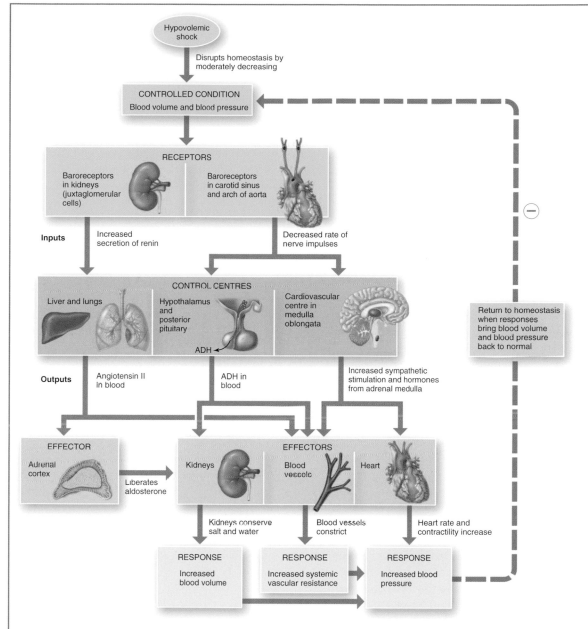

Figure 5.3 Restoration of blood pressure in hypovolaemic shock. *Source:* Tortora and Derrickson (2013).

Tissue Fluid Exchange

The main purpose of maintaining circulation within the cardiovascular system is to perfuse the tissues with oxygen and nutrients and then carry away their waste products. Despite the many types of blood vessels, this happens almost entirely at the level of the capillaries, which are uniquely adapted

for this function by having a very thin wall composed of a single layer of squamous (flat) epithelial cells and a basement membrane.

The exchange of soluble substances between the intravascular compartment and the interstitial compartment is known as *fluid exchange*. While individual substances may diffuse through the phospholipid bilayer driven by forces such as concentration gradients, a bulk of the exchange occurs through the movement of fluid from the intravascular compartment to the interstitial space, and vice versa. This exchange involves a filtration process driven by relative filtration pressures that were first described by British physiologist Ernest Starling in the late nineteenth century.

While many variables impact on this exchange, in its simplest format, the Starling Equation states that the net filtration pressure (NFP) is dependent on the difference between hydrostatic pressure (HP) and oncotic pressure (OP). HP is the outward pressure caused by fluid contained within a compartment, while OP is the inward pressure caused by osmotically active colloids present within each compartment (and is thus also known as *colloid osmotic pressure*).

The HP within the arterial end of capillaries is high, driven by the force provided by cardiac contractions. While the exact number may vary, the HP at this point could be approximated to about 36 mmHg. The OP is created by osmotically active particles that are too big to cross the phospholipid barrier. This is largely determined by the concentration of *albumin*, the most abundant plasma protein found in blood. Conventionally, the OP at the arterial end of a capillary is approximated at 25 mmHg. As the HP is 'pushing' fluid out and the OP is 'sucking' fluid in, they are in effect working against each other, with the NFP being the difference between the two forces. In the arterial end, based on the above approximations, this NFP would be in the region of 11 mmHg, thereby exerting an overall outward pressure. Fluid, and all soluble material dissolved within it, therefore moves predominantly from the intravascular compartment to the interstitial compartment, driven by this net outward pressure, in the arterial end of a capillary.

This flow of fluid from the intravascular compartment leads to a direct proportionate drop of the HP within the vascular compartment, without any change in the OP, as those particles (mainly albumin) do not cross the phospholipid bilayer. Again, while the exact number may vary from tissue to tissue, and within each point along the length of the capillary tree, conventionally this movement of fluid is contributory to a drop of HP to 15 mmHg by the time the blood reaches the venous end of the capillary. As there has been no change in OP (25 mmHg), this equates to an NFP of 10 mmHg

now being directed in towards to the intravascular space. This results in the bulk movement of fluid from the interstitial space to the intravascular space, again carrying all material, including tissue waste products that are dissolved within them, as long as they are small enough to filter through the endothelial cell walls.

Even considering the extremely simplified explanation above, it is evident that the NFPs at the arterial end (11 mmHg) and the venous end (10 mmHg) of the capillaries do not completely cancel each other out. In fact, about 15% of the volume of fluid filtered out of the arterial end does not return to the venous end of the capillary, thereby creating a potential accumulation of fluid in the extravascular fluid compartment, a phenomenon known as *oedema*. This problem is, however, averted by the presence of the lymphatic vessels, which works as a drainage system returning the excess fluid and other material that cannot enter capillaries to the main vascular compartment.

Clinical Relevance

Hypertension is a common longstanding condition characterised by persistent elevation of the BP. Although usually asymptomatic, hypertension is a risk factor for coronary heart disease, stroke, chronic kidney disease, peripheral vascular disease, and loss of vision. Elective dental treatment should be carried out only when hypertension is well controlled to reduce the risk of bleeding during dental surgical procedures. Moreover, care is required during the administration of vasoconstrictors containing local anaesthetic, such as adrenaline, to avoid any elevation of the BP.

Vasovagal fainting is the commonest medical emergency observed during dental treatment. Loss of consciousness may result from reduced venous return and consequent cerebral ischaemia (Chapter 22).

Postural (orthostatic) hypotension is characterised by a sudden fall in BP when standing up from a sitting or lying position. Causes include autonomic neuropathy as seen in diabetes (Chapter 18), medications (antihypertensives, recreational drugs, etc.), pregnancy (Chapter 20), and Addison's disease (Chapter 17). Patients receiving dental treatment in a supine position are particularly susceptible to postural hypotension when standing up, which may lead to fainting.

Migraine is a severe unilateral recurring headache associated with dilatation of the cerebral arteries and may be accompanied by nausea, photophobia, phonophobia, and difficulties in speech.

Temporal arteritis is an autoimmune condition which leads to inflammation of the temporal blood vessels and leads to severe facial pain affecting the temporal region. Similar involvement of the ophthalmic artery may lead to permanent blindness.

Reference

Tortora, G.J. and Derrickson, B. (2013). Principles of Anatomy and Physiology. Hoboken, NJ: Wiley.

Further Reading

Khan Academy (2018a). Arteries vs. veins: What's the difference? https://www.youtube.com/watch?v=7b6LRebCgb4 (accessed 1 May 2018).

Khan Academy (2018b). Arteries, arterioles, venules, and veins. https://www.youtube.com/watch?v=iqRTd1NYpU (acccessed 1 May 2018).

Kierszenbaum, A.L. and Tres, L.L. (2016). *Histology and Cell Biology: An Introduction to Pathology*, 4e. Philadelphia: Elsevier.

Sherwood, L. (2013). *Human Physiology: From Cells to Systems*, 8e. Boston: Cengage Learning.

Sherwood, L. (2016). The blood vessels and blood pressure. In: *Human Physiology: From Cells to Systems*, 9e, 335–379. Boston: Cengage Learning.

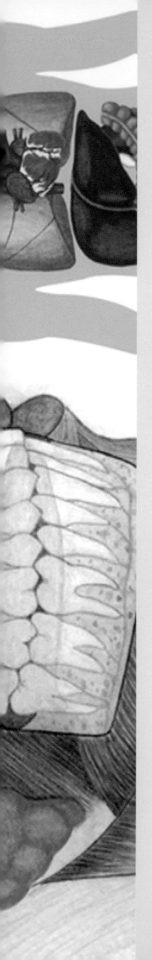

PART IV

Respiratory System

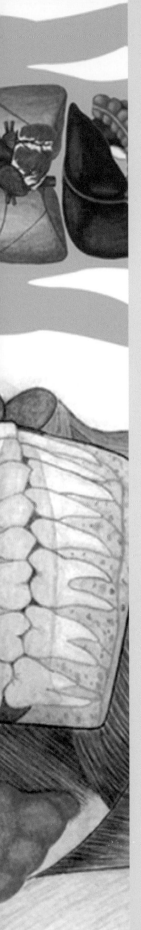

CHAPTER 6

Mechanics of Respiration

Feisal Subhan, Kamran Ali, and Elizabeth Prabhakar

Key Topics

- Overview of the respiratory system
- Common disorders affecting the respiratory system

Learning Objectives

To demonstrate an understanding of the:

- Structure and functional organisation of the respiratory system
- Mechanics of gas exchange between the atmosphere and the lungs
- Common indices used to measure gas exchange during inspiration and expiration
- Common obstructive and restrictive airway diseases and their impact on provision of dental care

Introduction

The main function of the lungs is to provide oxygen (O_2) to the tissues and remove carbon dioxide (CO_2) from the tissues. The primary actions which fulfil this function are: the mechanics of breathing, gas exchange and transport, and the control of breathing. O_2 is needed by the mitochondria for oxidative metabolism, i.e. energy (ATP) production (internal respiration), and CO_2 is generated as a waste product.

Other functions of the lungs include acting as a route for water (H_2O) loss and heat elimination, maintaining the body's acid base balance, enhancing venous return via the respiratory pump, forming speech with expiratory bursts of airflow, defence against inhaled foreign matter, converting the hormone angiotensin I to angiotensin II by angiotensin converting enzyme (ACE), and removing or inactivating blood clots.

Essential Physiology for Dental Students, First Edition. Edited by Kamran Ali and Elizabeth Prabhakar.
© 2019 John Wiley & Sons Ltd. Published 2019 by John Wiley & Sons Ltd.
Companion website: www.wiley.com/go/ali/physiology

Organisation of the Respiratory System

The respiratory system is divided into the upper and lower respiratory tracts. The upper tract includes the nasal cavity, pharynx, and larynx, while the lower tract comprises the trachea, bronchi, and the bronchial tree terminating in air sacs or alveoli. The lungs are located in the thorax and are surrounded by the pleural membrane, which contains a small amount (5 ml) of lubricating pleural fluid. The pleura is composed of two layers: the inner or parietal pleura lines the lungs, while the outer or visceral pleura connects the lungs to the rib cage, which protects the thorax and helps with respiratory movements. The right lung has three lobes, while the slightly smaller left lung has only two lobes as space is taken up by the pericardium. Within the lungs, each branching sequence of the bronchial tree is given a generation number. The dichotomy of the trachea into two main

bronchi is generation number 1. At the last generation number, approximately 23, an abundance of alveoli are found (Figure 6.1). There are an estimated 500 million alveoli in our lungs. The respiratory zone starts after generation number 17, as these terminal respiratory units allow diffusion of gas across their membranes. The region superior to this is called the *conducting zone*, as the primary function of these airways is to conduct air. In terms of cell histology, trachea and bronchi have cartilage and ciliated columnar epithelium. Smooth muscle and goblet cells are also present. The start of the respiratory zone is lined by squamous epithelium which have fewer cilia and smooth muscle and almost no goblet cells or cartilage. The numbers of alveoli increase till generation number 23. The alveoli are composed of two types of cells. Type 1 alveolar cells, which are flat in shape, have few organelles and have a supportive function. Type 2 alveolar cells secrete surfactant, an important phospholipoprotein. Phagocytic alveolar macrophages

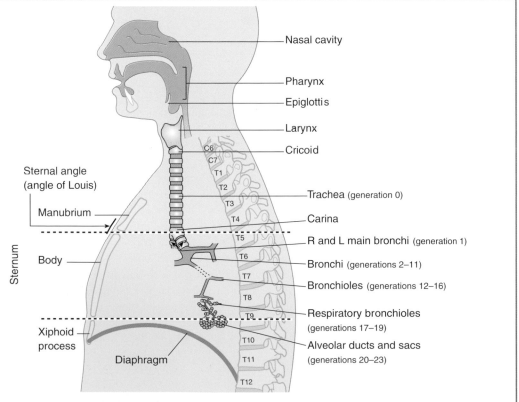

Figure 6.1 The airway passages, with their generation number, in relation to other structures in the thorax. *Source:* Ward et al. (2015).

are also present, and they keep the alveoli clear of harmful debris and microorganisms.

Lung Volumes and Capacities

There are four volumes and four capacities in the lung. The addition of two or more volumes forms capacities (Figure 6.2), e.g. functional residual capacity (FRC) = expiratory reserve volume (ERV) + residual volume (RV).

The lung volumes (Table 6.1) are determined by several factors, primarily height, age, gender, and ethnicity. Ethnicity can affect values by up to 15%, so specific reference values are used for different ethnic populations. Respiratory diseases can be classified as either obstructive, where bronchoconstriction results in altered airflow and airway resistance (R_{aw}), or restrictive, where the functional volume of the lungs decrease. An important measure of airway

obstruction is the forced expiratory volume in one second (FEV_1), which is the volume of air forcefully exhaled after starting from a maximal inspiration (TLC). In the clinic, a spirometer is used to measure slow vital capacity (VC) and forced vital capacity (FVC) manoeuvres. Figure 6.3 shows the FEV_1 and how it relates to the FVC in obstructive airways diseases, e.g. chronic obstructive pulmonary disease (COPD) and asthma. Spirometry measurements are important in quantifying the extent of disease impairment and are part of pre-operative evaluations to assess the effect of therapy and are also used to monitor environmental lung disease. Restrictive lung diseases are characterised by reduced TLC, measured by body plethysmography.

Respiratory Muscles

There are several muscles in the thorax and abdomen which are involved in altering lung volume during respiration. The main muscles and their functions are given in Table 6.2. The lungs primarily move in two ways: vertically, by the diaphragm and antero-posteriorly, by the action of the intercostals on the ribs. As is discussed in more detail in the next section, expiration is passive, owing to elastic recoil of the lung, and the expiratory muscles are for forced breathing (Figure 6.4), such as during exercise or performing a spirometric manoeuvre. The main inspiratory muscle is the diaphragm. The sternocleidomastoids, anterior serrati, and scalene muscles are often referred to as *accessory muscles of respiration*, as these are more active in forced breathing and also in disease.

Table 6.1 Typical lung volume and capacity values for a resting 70 kg male.

Lung volumes and capacities	Values (ml)
Tidal volume (V_T)	500
Inspiratory reserve volume (IRV)	3300
Expiratory reserve volume (ERV)	1700
Residual volume (RV)	1800
Functional residual capacity (FRC)	3500
Inspiratory capacity (IC)	3800
Vital capacity (VC)	5500
Total lung capacity (TLC)	7300

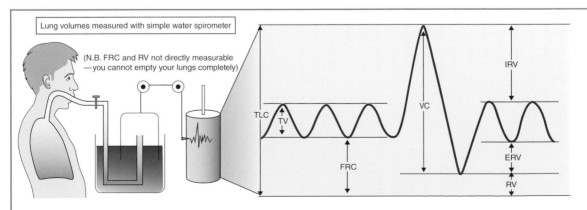

Figure 6.2 A water spirometer is used to produce a spirogram, which gives four lung volumes and four capacities. *Source:* Ward and Linden (2013).

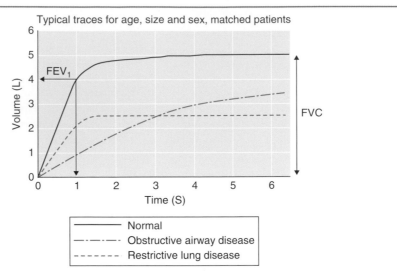

Figure 6.3 Measurements of FEV$_1$ and FVC in different disease states. *Source:* Ward and Linden (2013).

Table 6.2 The main muscles used in expiration and inspiration.

Expiratory muscles (forced breathing)	Inspiratory muscles
Abdominal muscles (move abdominal contents in and diaphragm upwards)	Diaphragm (pulls the lung downwards and increases vertical dimension of the thoracic cavity)
Internal intercostals (lowers ribcage)	External intercostals (lift ribcage)
	Sternocleidomastoids (lifts sternum)
	Anterior serrati (lift several ribs)
	Scalene muscles (lift first two ribs)

Mechanics of Pulmonary Ventilation

To understand the movement of air in and out of the lungs, we need to remember that the atmospheric air pressure (barometric pressure, or P_B) at sea level is normally 101.325 kPa (760 mmHg or 1 atm). The pressure exerted by a gas in a mixture of gases (like air) is the partial pressure (P). Although the pressure at the mouth is equivalent to P_B, by convention it is 0 kPa.

There are two other pressures to consider: the pleural pressure (P_{pl}), which is the pressure in the pleural space between the visceral and parietal pleurae, and the alveolar pressure (P_{alv}, or P_A), which is the pressure inside the alveoli. P_{pl} is negative at the beginning of resting inspiration. This is due to equal

and opposing forces on this membrane, as the lungs have a tendency to recoil or collapse, while the chest wall has a tendency to spring outwards. A continuous suction from the pleural membrane to the lymph also helps P_{pl} remain negative. When the glottis is open and there is no air flow, P_{alv} equals P_B, and by convention is 0 kPa. This occurs both at the beginning of inspiration and expiration, as shown in Figure 6.5.

Figure 6.5 also shows the change in the volume of air over inspiration and expiration. In a healthy person, this is normally about 0.5 l and is called the *tidal volume* (V_T). For air to enter the lung P_{alv} has to be negative and this occurs as the inspiratory muscles contract. These muscles include the diaphragm, which pull the lungs downward, while the external intercostal muscles raise the ribs projecting

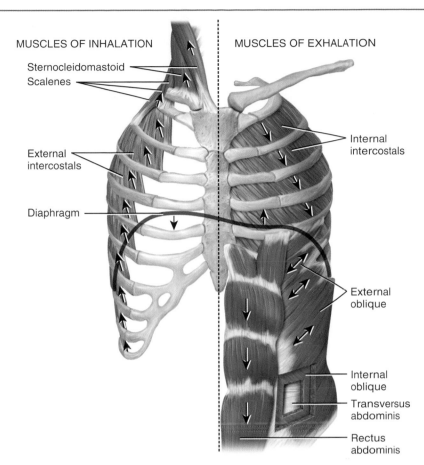

MUSCLES OF INHALATION   MUSCLES OF EXHALATION

Sternocleidomastoid

Scalenes

Internal
intercostals

External
intercostals

Diaphragm

External
oblique

Internal
oblique

Transversus
abdominis

Rectus
abdominis

Muscles of inhalation (left); muscles of exhalation (right);
arrows indicate the direction of muscle contraction

Figure 6.4 Respiratory muscles used for inhalation (inspiration) and exhalation (expiration). *Source:* Tortora and Derrickson (2013).

them forward, causing the sternum to move forward away from the spine. Inspiration is therefore active, in contrast to expiration, which is passive, as at rest it involves no muscles. After the inspiratory muscles contract, they stretch the lungs, creating a greater negative P_{pl}, this causes P_{alv} to go to $-0.1\,\text{kPa}$ and air is sucked in. A pressure of $-0.1\,\text{kPa}$ is enough to move 0.5 l of air (V_T) into the lungs.

From Figure 6.5, it can be seen that after air enters the lungs P_{alv} starts to approach $0\,\text{kPa}$ and simultaneously P_{pl} moves to its highest negative value. The difference between P_{alv} and P_{pl} is called the *transpulmonary* or *recoil pressure* ($P_L = P_{alv} - P_{pl}$) and is a measure of the forces that tend to collapse

the lung. At the beginning of inspiration $P_L = (0) - (-0.5) = +0.5\,\text{kPa}$, while at the beginning of expiration $P_L = (0) - (-0.75) = +0.75\,\text{kPa}$. This clearly indicates that at the beginning of expiration there is larger collapsing force and a greater recoil pressure, and this explains why expiration at rest is passive. Figure 6.6 shows a chronological flow chart of the steps needed for breathing to occur.

Lung Compliance

The extent to which the lungs expand for each unit of pressure is referred to as lung compliance (C_L). It is the ease of distention or stretching of the lung and

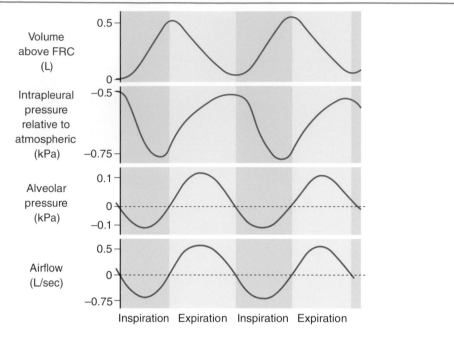

Figure 6.5 Volume, pleural pressure, alveolar pressure, and airflow changes during inspiration and expiration in a healthy subject at rest. *Source:* Ward et al. (2015).

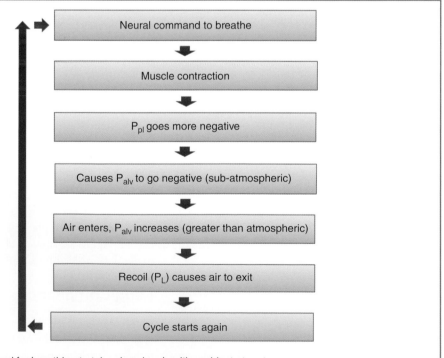

Figure 6.6 Steps required for breathing to take place in a healthy subject at rest.

can be calculated using the V_T, which is measured with a spirometer, and P_{pl}, which is determined by an oesophageal balloon catheter.

$$C_L = \frac{\Delta V}{\Delta P} = \frac{500(V_T)}{0.25\,(P_{pl}\,\text{change over inspiration})} \approx 2\,1\,\text{kPA}^{-1}$$

In lung fibrosis, which often occurs in occupational lung disease, C_L decreases, as the pressure needed to inflate the lungs to the same volume is greater. In emphysema, there is destruction of the structures supporting the alveoli, which is often due to smoking, resulting in loss of lung elasticity. In these patients, C_L increases, as the pressures needed for the same volume are less, owing to loss of elastic tissue. C_L increases with old age, too. C_L reflects the work done by the lungs. The overall work done in air-filled lungs can be divided into the elastic forces of lung tissues (elastin), the surface forces of surface tension (which make up two-thirds of total forces), lung tissue resistive work (collagen), and lastly airway resistance.

As mentioned above, most of the force needed to be overcome in breathing is surface tension. As an example, surface tension is seen when H_2O forms an interface with air. The H_2O molecules on the surface stick to each other by hydrogen bonding or cohesive forces. Surface tension can also be observed when a needle is gently placed on the surface of water in a glass container or in raindrops, where the strong attraction between H_2O molecules impedes their dispersion over great distances. However, surface tension can be disrupted by the addition of detergent, which breaks the hydrogen bonds holding the water molecules to lower surface tension. The lungs secrete *surfactant*, (which is a naturally occurring detergent containing dipalmitoylphosphatidylcholine), to decrease the surface tension inside alveoli. The benefits of pulmonary surfactant are to increase lung compliance and reduce recoil (to prevent early collapse). Both features which are altered in respiratory distress seen in preterm newborns, owing to a lack of surfactant production.

Normally, surfactant is secreted between the sixth and seventh month of gestation. It is more than just a detergent, as it also keeps the lungs dry and reduces the work done by the respiratory muscles during breathing. A lack of surfactant in preterm infants, owing to immature lungs or genetic reasons, results in infants making a big effort or forced inhalation to overcome the high surface tension. It is the most common lung disease affecting preterm infants. Synthetic surfactant is also available as a treatment option.

The maximum airflow resistance (R_{aw}) is found in the larger bronchioles and bronchi, at generation number 4 (refer to Figure 6.1). Smaller vessels have less R_{aw} primarily owing to an increase in their overall radius (i.e. their total cross-sectional area). The resistance to flow in vessels is $R_{aw} \propto 1/r^4$, where r is the radius of the tube. If the radius is halved, R_{aw} increases 16-fold. In asthmatics/COPD patients, R_{aw} increases during bronchoconstriction. R_{aw} is a good diagnostic and prognostic marker. Owing to Poiseuille's law, R_{aw} is lower during inspiration and higher during expiration, but in healthy lungs this is not a problem. However, in asthma, wheezing originates in the small airways, and they occur typically on expiration. During an asthmatic attack, these patients find expiration much more difficult than inspiration.

Clinical Relevance

COPD refers to a group of conditions characterised by irreversible narrowing of the airways, making expiration difficult. COPD includes conditions such as chronic bronchitis and emphysema and affects approximately three million patients in the UK. The main risk factor is smoking, but others include indoor air pollution (including using biomass fuel for cooking and heating), outdoor air pollution, occupational dusts or chemicals, and alpha-1 antitrypsin deficiency. Depending on the severity of the disease, several treatment planning modifications may be needed (e.g. shorter visits, avoiding treatment under conscious sedation and general anaesthesia). Patients may struggle to breathe when placed supine during dental treatment. Therefore, treatment is best carried out in an upright position. Treatment with steroids may cause complications in dental care, as described in Chapter 17.

Asthma is characterised by attacks of shortness of breath (breathlessness), coughing, and wheezing. Normally, this occurs by reversible airway narrowing and it affects 5.4 million patients in the UK. Most cases are atopic, where patients have a tendency to be sensitised to allergens. Dental patients with asthma will have similar treatment planning modifications as with COPD patients.

Tuberculosis (TB) is a bacterial infection that normally affects the lung, although it can affect other tissues or organs as well. Patients with an active infection can transmit the disease through air by coughing. Symptoms include chronic cough for more than three weeks, fever, weight loss, and fatigue. Elective dental work should be deferred until the patient is non-infectious and urgent work, should only be carried out with appropriate safety measures, such as infection control precautions and use of face masks by dental professionals.

References

Tortora, G.J. and Derrickson, B. (2013). *Principles of Anatomy and Physiology*. Hoboken, NJ: Wiley.

Ward, J.P.T. and Linden, R.W.A. (2013). *Physiology at a Glance*, 3e. Wiley.

Ward, J.P.T., Ward, J., and Leach, R.M. (2015). Lung mechanics. In: *The Respiratory System at a Glance*, 4e. Wiley-Blackwell.

Further Reading

Dr Najeeb Lectures (2018). Respiration: Physiology of respiratory system. https://www.youtube.com/watch?v=7dp5EoSEMY0 (accessed 1 May 2018).

Interactive respiratory physiology web resource. http://oac.med.jhmi.edu/res_phys/index.html (accessed 1 May 2018).

Pocock, G., Richards, C.D., and Richards, D.A. (2013). The respiratory system. In: *Human Physiology*, 4e, 449–491. Oxford: Oxford University Press.

Sherwood, L. (2013). *Human Physiology: From Cells to Systems*, 8e. Boston: Cengage Learning.

Sherwood, L. (2016). The respiratory system. In: *Human Physiology: From Cells to Systems*, 9e, 445–490. Boston: Cengage Learning.

CHAPTER 7
Gas Exchange and Transport

Feisal Subhan, Kamran Ali, and Elizabeth Prabhakar

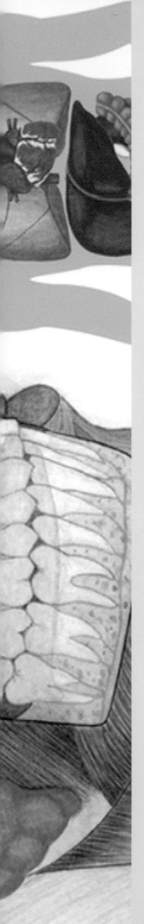

Key Topics

- Overview of gas exchange and transport
- Common disorders affecting gas transport

Learning Objectives

To demonstrate an understanding of the:

- Mechanisms of gas exchange between the lungs and blood
- Interpretation of common respiratory indices
- Transport of oxygen and carbon dioxide in the blood
- Relevance of common disorders of gas exchange and transport to the provision of dental care

Introduction

The exchange and transport of O_2 and CO_2 are vital to prevent hypoxia (low O_2) and hypercapnia (high CO_2). Various disease states can also affect the exchange and transport of these gases and consequently affect acid–base homeostasis (see next chapter). Gas exchange across the moist alveolar surfaces in the lungs takes place by passive diffusion, down the partial pressure gradients, i.e. from regions of high pressure to regions of low pressure.

Gas Diffusion

Air is a mixture of gases, as shown in Table 7.1. The pressure exerted by any one gas is a fraction of the total pressure and is referred to as the *partial pressure* (P). The pressure depends on the gas concentration and gas solubility. The total atmospheric pressure

Essential Physiology for Dental Students, First Edition. Edited by Kamran Ali and Elizabeth Prabhakar.
© 2019 John Wiley & Sons Ltd. Published 2019 by John Wiley & Sons Ltd.
Companion website: www.wiley.com/go/ali/physiology

(P_B) at sea level is 101.3 kPa (760 mmHg or 1 atm). Therefore, at sea level, the partial pressure of O_2 (PO_2) = 0.2098 × 101.3 = 21.3 kPa or 160 mmHg. The PCO_2, which is 0.30 mmHg, is negligible. Water (H_2O) vapour in the air reduces the gas per-

centages and their partial pressures, owing to dilution. Therefore, PO_2 will be lower by the time it reaches the alveoli, once the PH_2O (at 37 °C, is 6.27 kPa) is subtracted, i.e. PO_2 = 0.2098 × (101.3 − 6.27) = 19.9 kPa (see Figure 7.1).

A common 'trick question' is what is the percentage of O_2 at Mount Everest? The answer is the same as at sea level. What is lower is the P_B and therefore the PO_2, and this results in hypoxic conditions that normally only allow a mountain climber to ascend Mount Everest with the help of supplementary oxygen.

In the previous chapter, we discuss how air enters the lungs, now we need to understand how it diffuses across the alveolar-capillary membrane. Fick's Law determines the diffusion capacity for a gas, which is affected by four main factors: (i) *membrane thickness,*

Table 7.1 The approximate composition of various gases found in the atmosphere.

Gas	Approximate composition (%)
Nitrogen (N_2)	78.06
Oxygen (O_2)	20.98
Carbon dioxide (CO_2)	0.04
Helium and argon	0.92

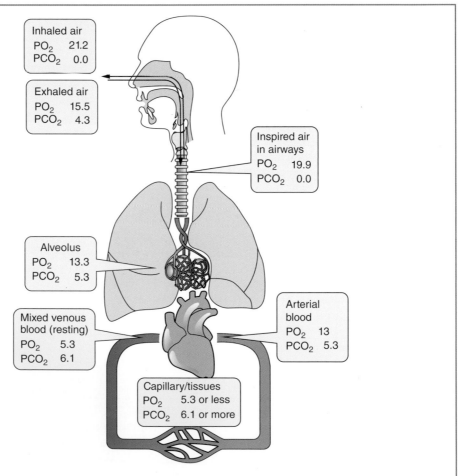

Figure 7.1 Partial pressures of O_2 and CO_2 across air passages and blood (in kPa). *Source:* Ward and Linden (2013).

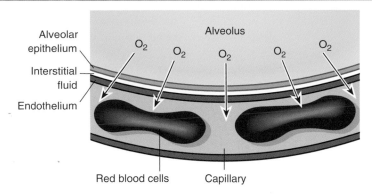

Figure 7.2 Diffusion of oxygen molecules across the alveolar-capillary membrane. *Source:* Ward, Ward, and Leach (2015).

which is directly proportional to the rate of diffusion. Thus, diffusion across the 0.6 μm thick alveolar-capillary membrane would be fast, (ii) surface area of the *membrane*, which is directly proportional to diffusion rate. The alveolar-capillary exchange surface is very large, spanning $70\,m^2$ with approximately 100 ml of capillary blood flowing through the capillary bed, (iii) *partial pressure gradient* (difference), the steeper the difference in partial pressure across the membrane, the faster the diffusion rate, and finally (iv) *diffusion coefficient or constant*, which depends on the gas solubility in blood and the molecular weight of the gas (Figure 7.2). The solubility of CO_2 is 23 times more than the solubility of O_2. When molecular weight is taken into account, the diffusion rate for CO_2 is 20.3, while it is 1.0 for O_2. This tends to suggest that CO_2 moves across the alveolar-capillary membrane much faster than O_2. However, the arteriovenous pressure gradient of O_2 is much greater than that of CO_2. This gradient is about 15% for CO_2 and 59% for O_2. Overall, therefore, O_2 and CO_2 have similar diffusion capacities.

In diseases, such as pulmonary oedema, fibrosis, and pneumonia, where the thickness of the alveolar-capillary membrane increases beyond 0.6 μm, a reduction in the rate of gas transfer occurs. In emphysema and lung collapse, the surface area of the membrane decreases and thus a decrease in rate of diffusion is seen in these pathological situations.

Respiratory Indices

Table 7.2 shows some physiological indices in healthy individuals.

Table 7.2 Normal physiological values for respiration in healthy individuals.

Indices	
Tidal volume (V_T)	0.5 l
Respiratory rate or frequency of breaths (f_R)	12 breaths min^{-1}
Expired ventilation ($\dot{V}_E$) = $V_T \times f_R$	6 l min^{-1}
Anatomical dead space (V_D)	0.15 l
Airflow or alveolar ventilation ($\dot{V}_A$) = f_R ($V_T - V_D$)	4.2 l min^{-1}
Blood flow, perfusion, or cardiac output ($\dot{Q}$)	5.5 l min^{-1}
Ventilation : Perfusion ratio = $\dot{V}/\dot{Q}$	0.8

$\dot{V}_E$ can reach 200 l min^{-1} during strenuous exercise. At rest, the total expired ventilation ($\dot{V}_E$; approximately 6 l min^{-1} in a healthy person) is not used in gas exchange, owing to the anatomical dead space (V_D), located in the nose, pharynx, larynx, and trachea.

Physiological dead space is associated with alveoli which are not functioning fully or have poor blood flow and is distinct from the anatomical dead space. Physiological dead space can result in poor gas exchange in certain respiratory diseases, e.g. a pulmonary embolus (an air bubble or blood clot which can block a pulmonary blood vessel).

Several factors may affect the ventilation/perfusion ($\dot{V}/\dot{Q}$) ratio. Owing to gravity, the apex of the lung has relatively less $\dot{Q}$, so $\dot{V}/\dot{Q}$ increases more than 0.8 (Figure 7.3). PO_2 will be more and likewise PCO_2 will be less here. However, at the base, $\dot{Q}$ is more relative to $\dot{V}_A$, so $\dot{V}/\dot{Q}$ falls below 0.8, resulting in a lower PO_2 and a greater PCO_2. A $\dot{V}/\dot{Q}$ ratio of 0.8 is an average value across the lung. In a patient with chronic obstructive pulmonary disease (COPD), smoking can often cause the alveoli distal to obstructed bronchioles to be poorly ventilated,

resulting in the $\dot{V}/\dot{Q}$ to approach 0. $\dot{V}/\dot{Q}$ scans are used in hospitals to detect any abnormal ventilation or perfusion in the lungs.

Transport of Oxygen in Blood

Haemoglobin (Hb) in the red blood cells transports O_2 and CO_2. Approximately, 97% of all O_2 transported in the blood is bound to Hb in the alveoli to form oxyhaemoglobin (HbO_2) which is delivered to the respiring tissues for aerobic respiration. The remaining 3% of O_2 is transported in a dissolved state in plasma and cells.

The relationship between PO_2 and the saturation of Hb gives rise to a characteristically shaped sigmoid (S-shaped) curve called the *oxygen dissociation curve* (Figure 7.4a). The curve demonstrates the affinity of Hb for O_2, or in other words the ease with which Hb can bind (associate) and release (dissociate) O_2 in the tissues.

Hb has the capacity to bind to four O_2 molecules (Figure 7.4b) and form HbO_2. Each O_2 molecule binds to one haem subunit in the Hb molecule. Each haem group has a central iron (Fe^{2+}) ion to which O_2 binds. A lack of Fe^{2+} causes anaemia, resulting in the inability of O_2 to bind to Hb. The curve is S-shaped because the binding of the first O_2

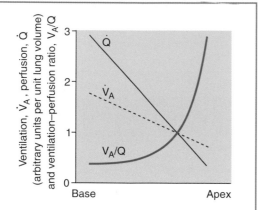

Figure 7.3 Changes in the $\dot{V}_A/\dot{Q}$ ratio, ventilation ($\dot{V}_A$), and perfusion (Q) taken across a healthy upright lung. *Source:* Ward, Ward, and Leach (2015).

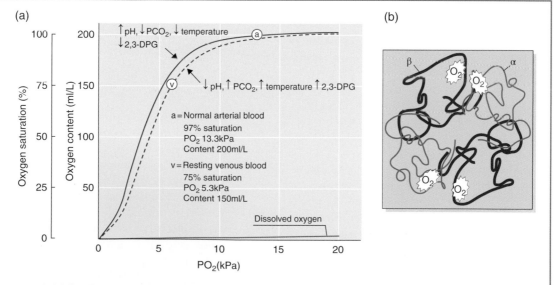

Figure 7.4 (a) O_2-Hb dissociation curve. The solid line is the standard oxygen dissociation curve and the dashed line shows four factors which shift the curve to the right. These are low pH, high PCO_2, high temperature, and high 2,3-DPG; (b) the Hb molecule showing the four haem subunits, with attached O_2 molecules. *Source:* Ward, Ward, and Leach (2015).

molecule makes it easier for the next O_2 to bind to Hb and so on, thus called *cooperative binding*.

Saturation of Hb is commonly expressed as a percentage. In normal arterial blood, saturation of Hb with O_2 is as high as 97% and PO_2 is as high as 13.3 kPa. In resting venous blood, saturation of Hb drops to 75%, owing to the low PO_2 of 5.3 kPa.

Factors Affecting Oxygen Dissociation Curve

Several factors affect the oxygen-dissociation curve, including pH, PCO_2, temperature, and 2,3-diphosphoglycerate (2,3-DPG), a metabolic by-product of glycolysis. A drop in the blood's pH (acidosis) or an increase in PCO_2, temperature, and 2,3-DPG shifts the curve to the right, which translates into a lower affinity of Hb to O_2, and release of O_2 into tissues. Exercise is one such stimulus that can shift all four factors so the curve shifts rightwards. Conversely, an increase in the blood's pH (alkalosis) or a decrease in PCO_2, temperature, and 2,3-DPG shifts the curve to the left, which translates into a higher affinity of Hb to O_2. This facilitates oxygenation of blood in the lungs.

Foetal Hb has a slightly different protein structure and a much higher affinity for O_2. This offers a benefit of allowing the foetus the ability to extract oxygen more effectively from maternal Hb.

The transport of O_2 can be adversely affected by hypoxia, anaemia, or ischaemia. On the other hand, *illegal blood doping* in athletes can increase the oxygen-carrying capacity, owing to a greater number of red blood cells.

Transport of Carbon Dioxide in Blood

CO_2 is transported in three forms in the blood: a small percentage (7%) is dissolved in plasma and cells, while 23% is transported bound to Hb as carbaminohaemoglobin ($HbCO_2$). Deoxygenated Hb has a higher affinity for CO_2 relative to oxygenated Hb (Haldane effect). The largest proportion of CO_2 (70%) is transported as bicarbonate (HCO_3^-) ions. Upon entering the red blood cells (RBCs), CO_2 combines with H_2O to form carbonic acid, a reaction catalysed by the enzyme carbonic anhydrase (CA). Carbonic acid dissociates rapidly to form $HCO3^-$ and H^+. The H^+ ion is buffered by the reduced Hb which is available after the release of O_2. This prevents a drop in blood pH (Chapter 13).

$$CO_2 + H_2O \xrightleftharpoons{Carbonic\ anhydrase} H_2CO_3 \rightleftharpoons HbH^+ + HCO_3^-$$

$$Hb + H^+ \rightleftharpoons HbH^+$$

HCO_3^- leaves the RBC via a HCO_3^-/Cl^- ion exchanger. This Cl^- shift results in an RBC Cl^- concentration greater in venous blood than in arterial blood (Figure 7.5).

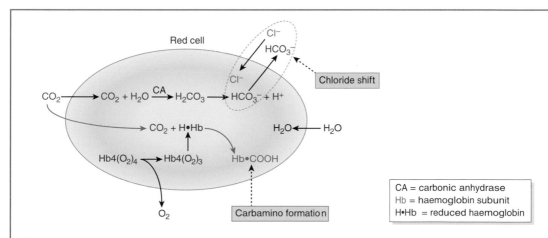

Figure 7.5 A red blood cell showing the transport mechanisms for CO_2. *Source:* Ward and Linden (2013).

Upon reaching the lungs, the venous blood is exposed to O_2 and the events are reversed, as shown in the following equation:

$$O_2 + HbH^+ + HCO_3^- \leftrightarrow HbO_2 + H_2O + CO_2$$

The CO_2 is eliminated in the exhaled air and O_2 combines with Hb to oxygenate the blood leaving the lungs.

Clinical Relevance

Airway protection during dental treatment is essential to avoid accidental displacement of dental materials, broken tooth fragments, and small instruments. Foreign body aspiration (FBA) may lead to respiratory obstruction and/or aspiration pneumonia, which can be potentially fatal, and often warrants removal with a bronchoscope. The right bronchus is wider, shorter, and more horizontal than the left bronchus; therefore, more FBA occurs in the right bronchus. Particular care is required in patients at extremes of age and those with neurocognitive disability. Use of barriers such as a rubber dam and physical protection with appropriate instruments and high-volume suction must be employed appropriately to prevent FBA during dental treatment.

Hypoxia is deficiency of oxygen. There are four classical types of hypoxia, which are important to understand as oxygen therapy differs for each. Hypoxic hypoxia occurs when partial pressure of O_2 in arterial blood (PaO_2) is reduced, for example at high altitude and in conditions such as asthma or pneumonia. Clinically, it is the most common type of hypoxia and administration of oxygen is beneficial (except where significant venous-to-arterial shunting takes place). Anaemic hypoxia is found when PaO_2 is normal, but Hb amounts are low and oxygen therapy is of limited use in these patients. Stagnant hypoxia is when Hb and PaO_2 are normal, but blood flow is diminished and oxygen therapy is again of limited use here. Histotoxic hypoxia is where O_2 delivery is normal, but, owing to a toxic substance, e.g. cyanide, tissues cannot utilise O_2. As with the two previous types of hypoxia, histotoxic hypoxic patients will have a limited benefit of oxygen therapy.

Cyanosis is a bluish discolouration of Hb and develops when there is a significant amount of reduced Hb in the blood. This can be noticed in the skin and mucous membranes and is often seen in patients with cardiopulmonary disease.

Carbon monoxide (CO) *poisoning* may result from several causes. CO has 210 times greater affinity for Hb than oxygen. It is a colourless, odourless gas and, if high enough, can result in CO poisoning and eventually death. Once bound to Hb, it forms carboxyhaemoglobin (COHb) and results in a cherry-red colour; it disassociates very slowly.

References

Ward, J.P.T. and Linden, R.W.A. (2013). *Physiology at a Glance*, 3e. Wiley.

Ward, J.P.T., Ward, J., and Leach, R.M. (2015). Lung mechanics. In: *The Respiratory System at a Glance*, 4e. Wiley-Blackwell.

Further Reading

Ball, W.C., Jr. (2018). Interactive respiratory physiology. http://oac.med.jhmi.edu/res_phys/index.html (accessed 1 May 2018).

Hasudungan, A. (2018). Control of respiration. https://www.youtube.com/watch?v=9j6BpanhpKY (accessed 1 May 2018).

Pathway Medicine (2018). Respiratory physiology. http://www.pathwaymedicine.org/respiratory-physiology (accessed 1 May 2018).

Pocock, G., Richards, C.D., and Richards, D.A. (2013). The respiratory system. In: *Human Physiology*, 4e, 449–491. Oxford: Oxford University Press.

Sherwood, L. (2013). *Human Physiology: From Cells to Systems*, 8e. Boston: Cengage Learning.

Sherwood, L. (2016). The respiratory system. In: *Human Physiology: From Cells to Systems*, 9e, 445–490. Boston: Cengage Learning.

CHAPTER 8
Control of Breathing

Feisal Subhan and Kamran Ali

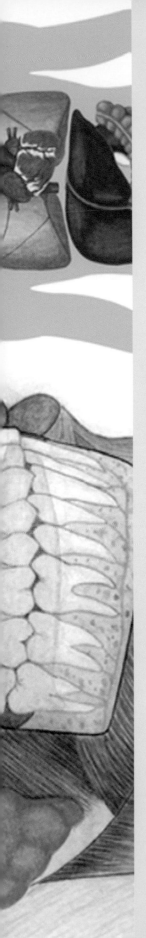

Key Topics

- Overview of the central and peripheral control of breathing
- Relevant disorders of breathing

Learning Objectives

To demonstrate an understanding of the:
- Organisation and functions of the neural respiratory centres
- Role of central and peripheral chemoreceptors
- Relevance of obstructive sleep apnoea to dental professionals

Introduction

Control of breathing is necessary so we can breathe enough to ensure maximum oxygen saturation of haemoglobin and also keep the work of breathing to a minimum. Additionally, carbon dioxide (CO_2) levels need close regulation, as changes can affect the pH of blood. If $\dot{V}_E$ is doubled, CO_2 decreases and it causes arterial pH to rise to 7.6, from a normal of 7.4. If $\dot{V}_E$ is halved, CO_2 levels increase, and pH falls to 7.2. Finally control of breathing allows us to 'override' the automatic reflex breathing in certain circumstances such as blowing, breath holding, swimming, and speech, etc.

Peripheral and Central Chemoreceptors

Peripheral and central chemoreceptors play an important role in the control of breathing. Peripheral chemoreceptors are found in the aortic and carotid bodies (Figure 8.1a). The carotid bodies have a very high blood flow and are the primary peripheral chemoreceptors.

Essential Physiology for Dental Students, First Edition. Edited by Kamran Ali and Elizabeth Prabhakar.
© 2019 John Wiley & Sons Ltd. Published 2019 by John Wiley & Sons Ltd.
Companion website: www.wiley.com/go/ali/physiology

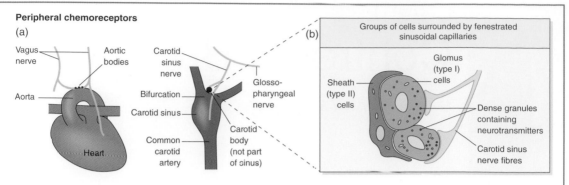

Figure 8.1 (a) Anatomical location of the carotid and aortic bodies. (b) Histology of the carotid body. *Source:* Ward, Ward, and Leach (2015).

They contain type I glomus and type II cells (Figure 8.1b); the latter have a supporting function.

Type I glomus cells release neurotransmitters, including catecholamines, when stimulated by hypoxia, and this results in afferent nerve action potentials. They also respond to increased concentrations of CO_2 and H^+ (hydrogen ion); although their primary response is hypoxia. If the peripheral chemoreceptors are denervated, approximately 30% of the response to increased CO_2 and H^+ levels, and most of the hypoxic response is lost. The glomus cells specifically respond to dissolved O_2 in blood, so carbon monoxide (CO) poisoning would not result in any afferent nerve firing. Only when PaO_2 (partial pressure of oxygen in arterial blood) levels fall to below 7 KPa does afferent nerve firing result in a significant increase in the $\dot{V}_A$ (Figure 8.2). Normal PaO_2 levels are approximately 13.3 KPa.

Central chemoreceptors, which are located in the medulla oblongata (Figure 8.3), contribute to ventilation even when carotid and aortic bodies are denervated. Central chemoreceptors are very sensitive to changes in H^+ concentration in the cerebrospinal fluid (CSF), which in turn are affected by arterial blood PCO_2 and pH.

Although CO_2, HCO_3^-, and H^+ all cross the blood–brain barrier, CO_2 has a higher permeability across a lipid bilayer, as it is a small, uncharged molecule. HCO_3^- and H^+, on the other hand, are ions and have a lower permeability. Therefore, CO_2 passes across the blood–brain barrier better than H^+, hence PCO_2 has a stronger ventilatory response than pH. Once a CO_2 molecule has diffused across into the CSF, it is hydrated and forms carbonic acid, which dissociates quickly to raise the H^+ ion concentration. An increase in PCO_2 (e.g. from an increased metabolism) increases $\dot{V}_A$. This is a negative feedback homeostatic mechanism, whereby the increased $\dot{V}_A$ would eventually blow off CO_2 and bring the PCO_2 level back to normal levels. Therefore, the medullary chemoreceptors are more sensitive to an increase in PCO_2 relative to an increase in H^+.

Neurons from both the peripheral and the central chemoreceptors can excite the neural respiratory centres. Only when PO_2 falls to very low levels does the system really respond. So, near the physiological range of blood gases, PCO_2 is a more important controller on a day-to-day basis.

Neural Respiratory Centres

The neural respiratory centres are found in the brainstem and are located bilaterally in the medulla oblongata and pons (Figure 8.4). The main areas which are responsible for automatic control of our breathing are the:

• Dorsal respiratory group (DRG) – which contains inspiratory neurons.
• Ventral respiratory group (VRG) – which contains inspiratory and expiratory neurons.
• Pre-Bötzinger complex (pre-BÖTC) – which has pacemaker cells and is found in the ventrolateral medulla (part of the VRG).
• Pneumotaxic centre or pontine respiratory groups – which alters the rate and pattern of breathing.

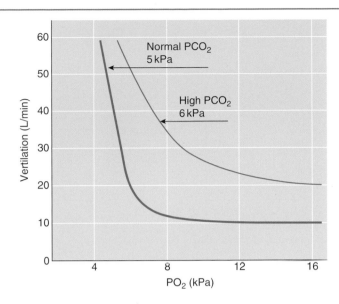

Figure 8.2 The relationship between PaO_2 and $\dot{V}_A$, while $PaCO_2$ remains constant and also when $PaCO_2$ is raised. *Source:* Ward and Linden (2013).

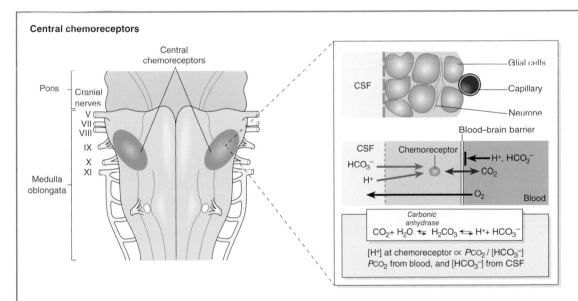

Central chemoreceptors

Figure 8.3 Anatomical location, histology, and biochemistry of the central chemoreceptors. *Source:* Ward, Ward, and Leach (2015).

It is important to note that inspiratory and expiratory neurons are spread across the medulla. Voluntary higher centre control can override the involuntary automatic control, e.g. during breath holding.

The pre-BÖTC is the basic rhythm generator, and efferent signals from here cause phrenic motor neurons to stimulate the diaphragm for inspiratory activity. The pre-BÖTC receives input from both the DRG and the VRG. Lesions of these two groups

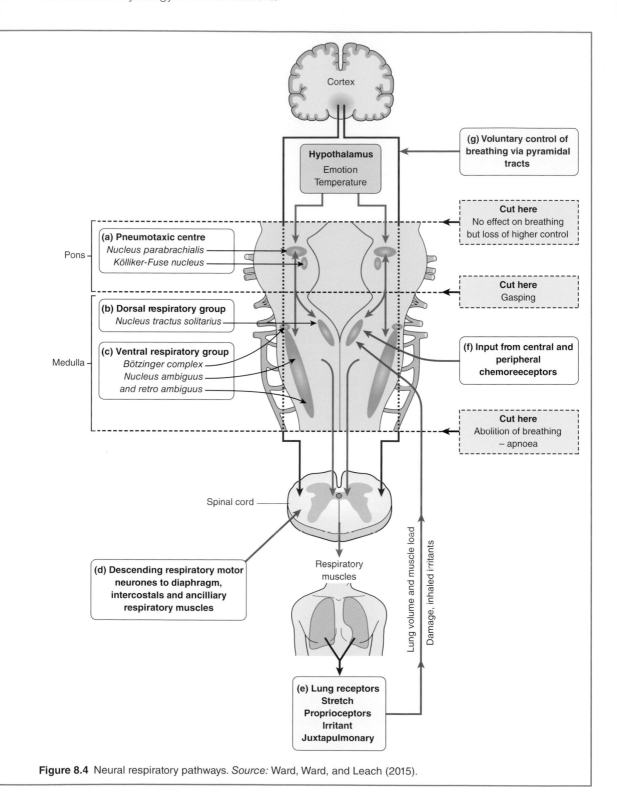

Figure 8.4 Neural respiratory pathways. *Source:* Ward, Ward, and Leach (2015).

do not stop respiration, but damage to the pre-BÖTC will. Most DRG neurons are in the nucleus tractus solitarius (NTS). The IXth (glossopharyngeal) and Xth (vagus) cranial nerves' sensory input reaches the NTS, carrying afferent information from chemoreceptors, baroreceptors, lung receptors, and proprioceptors. These afferents affect respiration. VRG neurons are found in the nucleus ambiguus and nucleus retroambiguus. At rest, VRG neurons are usually inactive. But, they are active at high rates of ventilation. They are especially important for abdominal muscle contraction in expiration. Reciprocal innervation at the spinal level prevents both the inspiratory and expiratory muscles from being contracted simultaneously. If a lesion occurs in the pontine respiratory groups, breathing becomes slow and deep (gasping-like; Figure 8.4). The exact function of these neurons is still not fully clear.

Peripheral Receptors

The airways and lungs are innervated by various receptors. These include the cough receptors, stretch receptors, and C-fibres. Cough receptors are rapidly adapting receptors and are found in epithelial cells of the upper airways and trachea-bronchial tree. They are stimulated by irritants such as dust, smoke, or chlorine gas and result in cough, bronchoconstriction, and mucus secretion. Stretch receptors are slowly adapting receptors and are found in the smooth muscle of small and large airways. They are thought to be more important during infancy and this reflex protects the lung from over-inflation. This is also known as the *Hering–Breuer reflex*, and these receptors cause cessation of inspiration once stimulated. C-fibres are found in the bronchial and pulmonary blood vessels and interstitium. Their stimulus includes pulmonary emboli or oedema, and the effect is an apnoea followed by tachypnoea and possibly dyspnoea. Studies on patients with lung transplants show that their patterns of breathing are normal at rest, indicating that intrapulmonary receptors may not play a vital role in regulation of breathing at rest.

Clinical Relevance

Obstructive sleep apnoea (OSA) is one of a group of conditions that fall under the umbrella term *sleep-disordered breathing*. This includes central sleep apnoea and obesity hypoventilation syndrome. OSA is the most common of all these conditions. All these conditions affect breathing during sleep. Risk factors for OSA include obesity, short mandible, macroglossia (large tongue), and pharyngeal narrowing. For example, Down's syndrome patients are at risk of developing OSA. Dental professionals may be able to identify anatomical features which increase the risk of OSA and refer patients appropriately. Moreover, dentists may be able to provide suitable oral appliances to patients with OSA and reduce its severity. OSA commonly results in snoring. It has been estimated that up to 20% of all adults have mild OSA. OSA increases the risk for stroke, coronary heart disease, diabetes mellitus, and increased accidents (including motor vehicle collisions).

References

Ward, J.P.T. and Linden, R.W.A. (2013). *Physiology at a Glance*, 3e. Wiley.

Ward, J.P.T., Ward, J., and Leach, R.M. (2015). Lung mechanics. In: *The Respiratory System at a Glance*, 4e. Wiley-Blackwell.

Further Reading

Ball, W.C., Jr. (2018). Interactive respiratory physiology. http://oac.med.jhmi.edu/res_phys/index.html (accessed 1 May 2018).

Hasudungan, A. (2018). Control of respiration. https://www.youtube.com/watch?v=9j6BpanhpKY (accessed 1 May 2018).

Pocock, G., Richards, C.D., and Richards, D.A. (2013). The respiratory system. In: *Human Physiology*, 4e, 449–491. Oxford: Oxford University Press.

Sherwood, L. (2016). The respiratory system. In: *Human Physiology: From Cells to Systems*, 9e, 445–490. Boston: Cengage Learning.

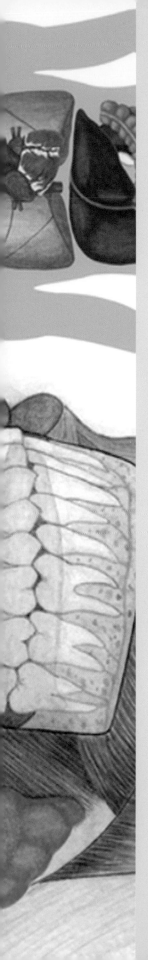

PART V

Gastrointestinal System (GIT)

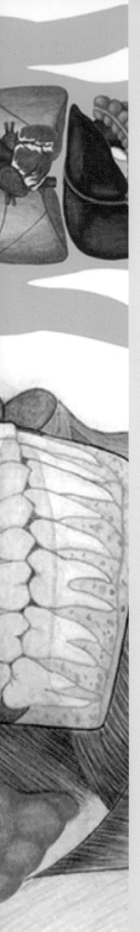

CHAPTER 9
GIT Movements

Kamran Ali

Key Topics

- Overview of movements of the gastrointestinal tract
- Common disorders of gastrointestinal movements

Learning Objectives

To demonstrate an understanding of the:
- Structure and functional organisation of the gastrointestinal tract
- Mechanisms and control of mastication and deglutition
- Mechanisms controlling the motor functions of the stomach, and small and large intestines
- Common disorders of gastrointestinal movements and their impact on oral and dental health

Introduction

The gastrointestinal tract (GIT) extends from the mouth to the anus and has several associated glands which contribute to a variety of secretions (Figure 9.1). The GIT is responsible for the breakdown, digestion, and absorption of food and excretes the waste from the body. Movements of the GIT propel ingested food from the oral cavity to the large intestine and help mixing of the food with GIT secretion to facilitate digestion and absorption of food.

The wall of the GIT from the lower oesophagus down to the anus is composed of four layers: mucosa, submucosa, muscularis, and serosa (Figure 9.2). The GIT is innervated by input from the somatic nervous system and autonomic nervous system. In addition, the GIT has an extensive local system of nerves, known as the *enteric nervous system*, which extends from the oesophagus to the terminal part of the large intestine. The enteric

Essential Physiology for Dental Students, First Edition. Edited by Kamran Ali and Elizabeth Prabhakar.
© 2019 John Wiley & Sons Ltd. Published 2019 by John Wiley & Sons Ltd.
Companion website: www.wiley.com/go/ali/physiology

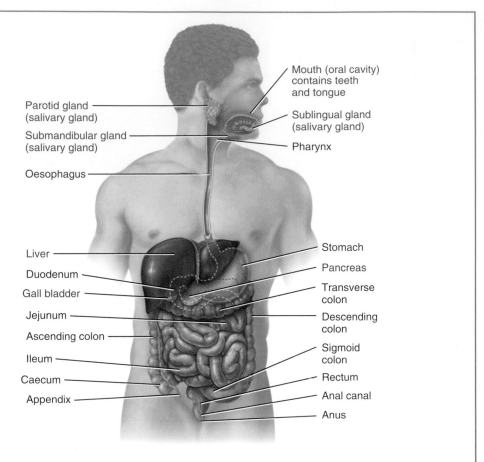

Figure 9.1 The gastrointestinal tract extends from the mouth to the anus. *Source:* Tortora and Derrickson (2013).

nervous system consists of two types of nerve plexuses: the *myenteric plexus* in the muscular layers of the GIT plays a role in controlling GIT movements and *Meissner's plexus* in the submucosa plays a role in controlling GIT secretions. Although the enteric nervous system is stimulated by the autonomic nervous system, it is also capable of functioning independently.

Mastication

Mastication or chewing is the first step in the process of digestion and serves to prepare the food for swallowing and its processing in the stomach and intestines. The teeth grind the food into smaller fragments, and this process is aided by saliva, which lubricates the food and helps in taste perception. The incisors cut and shear the food, the canines help in griping and tearing the food, while the premolars and molars provide a grinding action. The bite force depends on the number of teeth, volume, activity, and coordination of masticatory muscles. In fully dentate individuals, forces generated during mastication may be up to 50 pounds in the incisor region and 200 pounds in the molar region.

Mastication is initiated as a voluntary process and involves both sensory and motor nerve signals. Following ingestion of food, it is transported from the front of the mouth to the occlusal surfaces of the teeth to initiate a series of chewing cycles. Ingestion and mastication of food is aided by facial muscles, tongue, masticatory muscles (masseter, temporalis, lateral pterygoid, and medial pterygoid), and suprahyoid muscles (digastric, geniohyoid, mylohyoid, and stylohyoid).

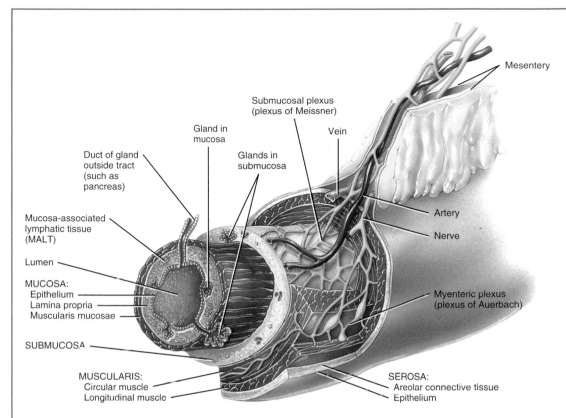

Figure 9.2 Layers of the gastrointestinal tract showing enteric nervous system. *Source:* Tortora and Derrickson (2013).

The muscles of mastication are controlled by the trigeminal nerve (V CN), and the masticatory reflexes are controlled by nuclei in the brainstem with input for the higher centres in the cerebral cortex, hypothalamus, and amygdala (appetite centres); it also has connections with the salivatory, gustatory, and olfactory nuclei. In addition, the mesencephalic nucleus of the trigeminal nerve receives proprioceptive input from the teeth (periodontal ligament), mandible, and temporomandibular joints (TMJ). These connections allow coordination of general sensory, proprioceptive, gustatory, salivatory, and olfactory reflexes with mastication.

The rhythmic contraction of the muscles controlling jaw opening and closure is determined by a central pattern generator located in the brainstem. The presence of food in the mouth initiates reflex inhibition of jaw-closing muscles (temporalis, masseter, and medial pterygoid) and activation of jaw-opening muscles (lateral pterygoid and suprahyoid muscles) allowing the mandible to drop. A stretch reflex follows and causes a rebound contraction of jaw-closing muscles allowing the teeth to contact the food again and the cycle is repeated. In addition to simple depression (opening) and elevation (closure) of the mandible, masticatory movements also involve protrusion, retraction, and side-to-side movements of the jaw. All jaw movements are ultimately translated at the TMJ.

Once initiated, mastication is largely a subconscious activity. Nevertheless, voluntary control is maintained, and mastication can be interrupted if the teeth encounter a hard object in the food, such as a stone or piece of bone. The number of chewing cycles depends on the texture, taste, temperature, and palatability of food. When the food has been chewed, it is termed a *bolus*. The tongue then pushes the bolus back towards the oropharynx to initiate swallowing.

Clinical Relevance

Bruxism is a parafunctional habit, often associated with physical or psychological stress. It is characterised by involuntary jaw clenching and grinding of teeth usually during sleep, though it may also be observed in the daytime. Bruxism may lead to *attrition*, a type of tooth surface loss involving the occlusal surfaces of posterior teeth and incisal edges of anterior teeth. In addition, bruxism may lead to hypertrophy of masticatory muscles, which is usually most conspicuous in the masseter muscles and results in facial asymmetry and/or a squarish appearance of the face. Moreover, bruxism may also lead to displacement and damage to the disc of the TMJ, which is often manifested by joint pain, clicking, and reduced mouth opening.

Advanced periodontal disease characterised by gross tooth mobility reduces masticatory efficiency. Similarly, loss of teeth, especially the molars, reduces masticatory efficiency and often warrants replacement with artificial teeth. Derangement of occlusion may result from facial trauma or improper restorative dentistry and causes reduced masticatory efficiency. The masticatory system has an ability to adapt to changes in food type or occlusion, loss of teeth, or to dental appliances, such as dentures.

Swallowing

Swallowing, or deglutition, allows the passage of food, drinks, and medicines from the oropharynx into the oesophagus and ultimately into the stomach. The pharynx is also a passage for breathing, and the act of swallowing lasts only a few seconds to ensure that breathing is interrupted for as short a time as possible. Swallowing involves a complex neuromuscular activity and is divided into three phases, namely oral, pharyngeal, and oesophageal (Figure 9.3).

Oral (Voluntary) Phase

Once the bolus of food has been prepared by mastication, it is voluntarily rolled back towards the oropharynx. This involves contraction of the orbicularis oris muscle allowing the lips to adduct and seal the oral cavity followed by elevation of the tongue. These movements allow the bolus to be pressed between the tongue and the palate, facilitating its transport towards the oropharynx.

Pharyngeal (Involuntary) Phase

This phase is involuntary and involves the transport of food from the oropharynx into the oesophagus. This phase usually lasts for up to six seconds and is accompanied by inhibition of breathing. The presence of food in the region of the palatoglossal and palatopharyngeal arches (tonsillar pillars) initiates a complex sequence of muscular contractions to accomplish the pharyngeal phase. These include:

- Elevation of the soft palate blocks the posterior nasal apertures, preventing entry of food into the nose.
- The palatopharyngeal arches are pulled medially, forming a narrow slit for the passage of food suitable for swallowing and at the same time preventing large pieces of food to go through.
- The pharynx along with the hyoid bone is pulled upwards and forwards by the pharyngeal and suprahyoid muscles.
- The larynx is pulled antero-superiorly, the vocal cords are approximated, and the epiglottis covers the laryngeal opening. These movements prevent entry of food into the larynx and trachea.
- The upper oesophagus (pharyngo-oesophageal) sphincter relaxes.
- Finally, the contraction of pharyngeal muscles propels the bolus down the pharynx into the oesophagus.

The muscular movements are controlled by the *swallowing centre* in the brainstem (pons and medulla). Afferent impulses to the swallowing centre are transmitted by the branches of the trigeminal and glossopharyngeal nerves. The efferent (motor) impulses to the muscles of the palate, pharynx, and oesophagus are transmitted by the trigeminal, pharyngeal plexus (glossopharyngeal, vagus, and accessory nerves), hypoglossal, and superior cervical nerves.

Oesophageal (Involuntary) Phase

This phase transports the food from the oesophagus into the stomach. The upper oesophagus walls contain striated muscles innervated by the glossopharyngeal (IX CN) and vagus (X CN). The lower two-thirds of the oesophageal walls contain smooth muscles and receive dual innervation from the local myenteric plexus as well as the vagus nerves.

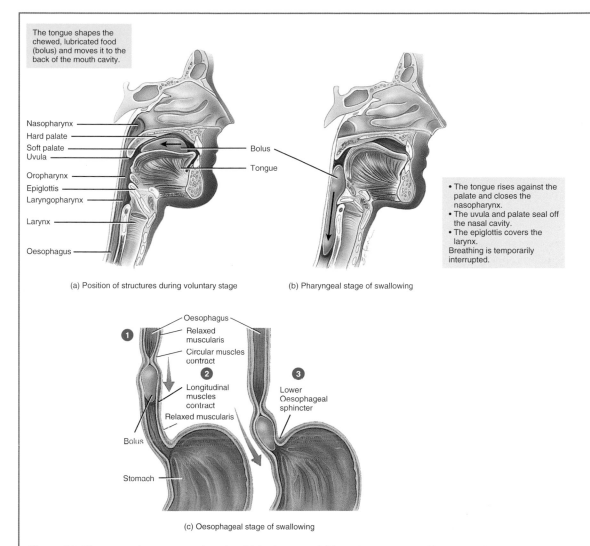

The tongue shapes the chewed, lubricated food (bolus) and moves it to the back of the mouth cavity.

Nasopharynx
Hard palate
Soft palate
Uvula
Oropharynx
Epiglottis
Laryngopharynx
Larynx
Oesophagus

Bolus
Tongue

• The tongue rises against the palate and closes the nasopharynx.
• The uvula and palate seal off the nasal cavity.
• The epiglottis covers the larynx.
Breathing is temporarily interrupted.

(a) Position of structures during voluntary stage

(b) Pharyngeal stage of swallowing

Oesophagus
❶ Relaxed muscularis
Circular muscles contract
❷ Longitudinal muscles contract
Relaxed muscularis
❸ Lower Oesophageal sphincter
Bolus
Stomach

(c) Oesophageal stage of swallowing

Figure 9.3 Diagrammatic representation of oral (a), pharyngeal (b), and oesophageal (c) phases of swallowing. *Source:* Tortora and Derrickson (2013).

The oesophageal phase is accomplished by continuation of the peristaltic wave generated in the pharynx and, when aided by gravity (upright position), allows the food to reach the stomach in five to eight seconds. If the bolus of food is too large for the primary peristaltic wave to transport the food down the oesophagus, secondary peristaltic waves are initiated, following the distension of the oesophageal walls. The secondary peristaltic waves are initiated by stimulation of the myenteric plexus as well as by efferent nerve fibres from the glossopharyngeal and vagus nerves.

The transmission of the peristaltic wave from the oesophagus to the stomach is preceded by relaxation of the lower oesophageal (gastro-oesophageal) sphincter allowing entry of the bolus into the stomach.

Clinical Relevance

Gastro-oesophageal reflux disease (GORD) is characterised by regurgitation of oesophageal and stomach contents into the oral cavity. Risk factors include pregnancy, obesity, smoking, incompetent lower oesophageal sphincter, and hiatus hernia. The latter is caused by protrusion of the stomach into the chest cavity due to a weakness in the diaphragm. GORD may lead to erosion of the dental hard tissues, as explained in Chapter 10.

Dysphagia, or difficulty in swallowing, may be associated with several conditions such as neurological disorders (head injury, stroke, dementia, Parkinsonism), cancer of the mouth and oesophagus, and GORD. Moreover, spreading oral infections may involve the pharynx and lead to dysphagia. Developmental anomalies of the palate, such as cleft palate, lead to difficulties in feeding and swallowing in infants. Feeding aids may be required until a surgical repair of the defects is undertaken.

The *gag reflex* is triggered by tactile stimulation soft tissues of the posterior tongue, soft palate, tonsillar regions, and pharynx. An intact gag reflex helps to prevent choking. Spillage of local anaesthetic agents in the mouth may lead to temporary impairment of gag reflex. Some individuals have *hypersensitive gag reflex* (HGR), which is activated by the presence of objects in the mouth. Dental instrumentation and dental impression-taking in individuals with HGR may be challenging because of persistent gagging.

Movements of the Stomach

The stomach is a hollow muscular organ that connects the oesophagus with the duodenum (small intestine). Entry of food from the oesophagus into the stomach is controlled by the lower-oesophageal sphincter, while the pyloric sphincter controls the passage of food from the stomach to the duodenum (Figure 9.4). The stomach is divided into several regions:

- *Cardia:* the region connecting the stomach with the lower oesophagus.
- *Fundus:* the superior curvature of the stomach.
- *Body:* the central region constituting the main bulk of the stomach.
- *Pylorus:* the lower region connecting the stomach with the duodenum.

The motor functions of the stomach include mixing of food with gastric secretions to form a semi-fluid mixture known as *chyme*, storage of food, and emptying of chyme into the small intestine.

Entry of food into the stomach distends its muscular wall and activates parasympathetic impulses which relax the stomach muscles, greatly increasing its capacity to accommodate large quantities of food. The volume of the stomach usually ranges from 1 to 1.5 l. but distension by food may increase it three- to fourfold.

Contractions of the stomach wall allow gastric secretions to mix with the food and turn it into a

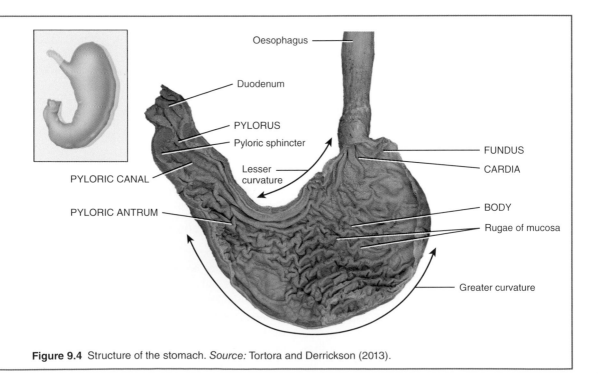

Figure 9.4 Structure of the stomach. *Source:* Tortora and Derrickson (2013).

semi-fluid mixture (chyme). When the chyme is ready to be emptied into the duodenum, the stomach contractions become five- to sixfold stronger, transforming into intense peristaltic waves often referred to as *pyloric pump*. Although highly variable, 50% of stomach contents are usually emptied in two to three hours. However, the total transit time of food in the stomach may be up to five hours.

The rate of emptying of chyme into the duodenum is controlled by gastric as well as intestinal factors. Gastric factors increase the activity of the pyloric pump, promoting emptying of the stomach. These include distension of the stomach wall by chyme, which stimulates the myenteric plexus and release of a hormone, *gastrin*, from the stomach mucosa. On the other hand, entry of chyme into the duodenum reduces stomach emptying. The rate of stomach emptying is reduced with increased volume and acidity of the duodenal chyme. In addition, presence of irritants and protein breakdown products in the duodenal chyme also reduce stomach emptying. These inhibitory reflexes are mediated by the local myenteric plexus, autonomic nerves, and several hormones including: *cholecystokinin* (released by the jejunum), *secretin* (released by the duodenum), and *gastric inhibitory peptide* or *glucose-dependent insulinotropic peptide* (released by the duodenum).

Movements of the Small Intestine

Th small intestine consists of duodenum, jejunum, and ileum and measures approximately 6 m (20 ft) in length and 2.5–3 cm (1 in.) in diameter (Figure 9.5). Its movements serve to mix and propel food. The presence of chyme causes segmental contractions of the small intestine at a rate of 8–12 contractions per minute. The contractions are generated by electrical slow waves generated in the intestinal wall and stimulation of the myenteric plexus. The small intestine is the main site of digestion and absorption of nutrients. The contractions help to mix the food with the intestinal secretions and spread the chyme against the intestinal mucosa for absorption. In addition to mixing, the contractions of the small intestine generate peristaltic waves which propel the food through the small intestine at a rate of 1 cm per minute. The peristaltic waves in the small intestine primarily represent continuation of the peristalsis generated by the myenteric plexus in the stomach. The intestinal peristalses are enhanced further by the presence of chyme, which distends the intestinal wall. Finally,

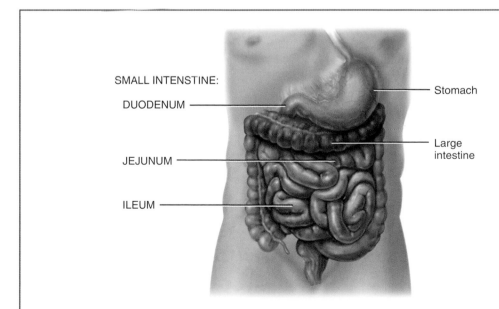

Figure 9.5 External anatomy of the small intestine (Anterior view). *Source:* Tortora and Derrickson (2013).

several hormones, such as gastrin, cholecystokinin, and insulin, also increase intestinal motility.

The emptying of chyme from the *ileum*, the terminal part of the small intestine into the colon, is controlled by the *ileocaecal sphincter* which lines the *ileocaecal valve* at the junction of terminal ileum and caecum. The ileocaecal valve also prevents the backflow of faecal contents from the colon into the small intestine. The transit time of chyme in the small intestine ranges from three to five hours, and its emptying into the caecum is facilitated by powerful contractions of the ileum (gastro-ileal reflex), relaxation of the ileocaecal sphincter and reflex feedback from the colon.

Movements of the Large Intestine

The large intestine, or colon, is an approximately 1.5 m long muscular tube. It consists of four parts: the ascending colon, the transverse colon, the descending colon, and the sigmoid colon. The ascending colon is connected to the ileum by an out pocketing of the large intestine, known as the *caecum*. The sigmoid colon leads to the rectum, which provides a route for expulsion of the faecal waste through defaecation (Figure 9.6).

The proximal parts of the colon (ascending and transverse colon) are primarily responsible for the absorption of salts and water, while the function of the distal half of the colon (descending and sigmoid colon) is to store faecal matter before it is emptied into the rectum.

The colon provides two types of movements. Firstly, *mixing movements* result from the periodic contractions of muscular wall of the colon and aid in the absorption of water and electrolytes in the chyme. Approximately 1.5- 2 l of chyme is emptied into the large intestine each day but only 100–200 ml is expelled as faeces. Secondly, propulsive or *mass movements* occur one to three times per day, especially in the morning. The mass movements are modified peristaltic movements characterised by a series of contractions lasting for 10–30 minutes and facilitate propulsion of the faecal matter into the rectum.

Normally, entry of intestinal contents into the rectum is prevented by the constriction of a thickened band of circular smooth muscle (*internal anal sphincter*), located between the sigmoid colon and rectum. Moreover, the *external anal sphincter*, located distal to the internal anal sphincter and surrounding the anus, prevents expulsion of faeces through the anus.

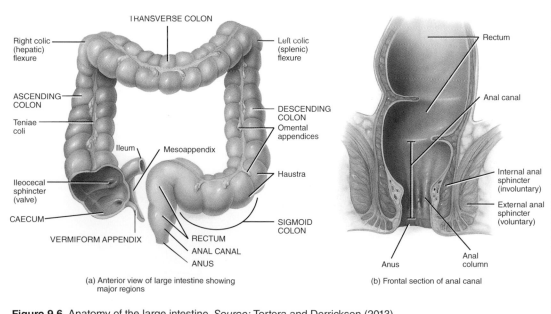

Figure 9.6 Anatomy of the large intestine. *Source:* Tortora and Derrickson (2013).

Mass movements force the faeces into the rectum leading to distension of the rectal walls. This stimulates peristalsis through the local myenteric plexus followed by activation of the parasympathetic fibres in the pelvic nerves. These nerve signals ultimately initiate the *defaecation reflex*, which involves inhibition of the internal anal sphincter (involuntary) and relaxation of the external anal sphincter (voluntary). In addition, the defaecation is aided by taking a deep breath, forced expiration against a closed glottis (Valsalva manoeuvre), and contraction of the abdominal muscles to force the expulsion of the faecal matter through the anus. Relaxation of the external anal sphincter is often accompanied by relaxation of the urethral sphincter and this explains why defaecation is often accompanied by simultaneous urination.

Clinical Relevance

Defaecation is largely under voluntary control except in infants and young children. Loss of voluntary control of defaecation and/or urination (incontinence) may result from diarrhoea; physical trauma, including surgical insults; inflammatory bowel disease; and psychological factors, such as fright.

Reference

Tortora, G.J. and Derrickson, B. (2013). *Principles of Anatomy and Physiology*. Hoboken, NJ: Wiley.

Further Reading

Campbell, J. (2018). Gastrointestinal anatomy and physiology. https://www.youtube.com/watch?v=w_54aqc8Des (accessed 1 May 2018).

Cork, A. (2018). Swallowing. https://www.youtube.com/watch?v=pNcV6yAfq-g (accessed 1 May 2018).

Hall, J.E. (2015). Chapter 63. In: *Guyton and Hall Textbook of Medical Physiology*, 12e. Elsevier.

Khan Academy (2018). Health and medicine advanced gastrointestinal physiology. https://www.khanacademy.org/science/health-and-medicine/gastro-intestinal-system/gastrointestinal-intro/v/meet-the-gastrointestinal-tract (accessed 1 May 2018).

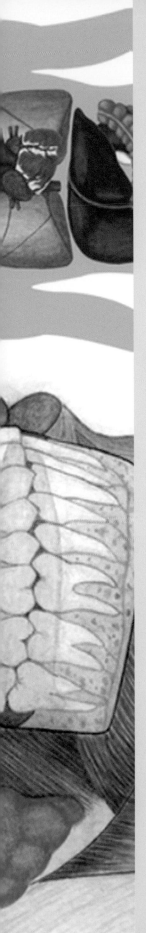

CHAPTER 10
GIT Secretions

Kamran Ali

Key Topics

- Overview of gastrointestinal tract secretions
- Common disorders of gastrointestinal secretions

Learning Objectives

To demonstrate an understanding of the:

- Composition, functions, and control of saliva, gastric juice, pancreatic juice, bile, and intestinal juice
- Common disorders of gastrointestinal secretions and their impact on oral and dental health

Introduction

The gastrointestinal (GIT) tract produces a variety of secretions which play a key role in the digestion of food. Moreover, the lining of the GIT contains millions of mucous glands which produce mucous. Mucous is a thick viscous secretion which helps in the lubrication of food, facilitates digestive movements, and protects the GIT lining from irritation by food and digestive secretions. The exocrine glands associated with the GIT secrete up to 7 l of fluid daily. In addition, 2.0–2.5 l of fluids are ingested each day. Apart from approximately 100 ml expelled in the faeces, the remaining fluid is reabsorbed in the intestines, reflecting the contribution of GIT to haemostasis. The secretions contain mucous, digestive enzymes, electrolytes, and other ingredients. The primary stimulus for secretions is the presence of food in different parts of the GIT. The neural control of GIT secretions is provided by the local (enteric) nervous system as well as the autonomic nervous system. Parasympathetic stimulation generally causes a marked increase in the rates of secretion in most parts of the GIT. Although

Essential Physiology for Dental Students, First Edition. Edited by Kamran Ali and Elizabeth Prabhakar.
© 2019 John Wiley & Sons Ltd. Published 2019 by John Wiley & Sons Ltd.
Companion website: www.wiley.com/go/ali/physiology

sympathetic stimulation causes a mild to moderate increase in secretions, it also causes vasoconstriction in the glands. Sympathetic vasoconstriction may reduce the effect of parasympathetic or hormonal secretion and indirectly lead to a reduction in secretions. In addition, several hormones also influence the rate and character of GIT secretions.

Saliva

Saliva is produced by exocrine glands known as *salivary glands*. These include three pairs of major salivary glands – i.e. the parotid, submandibular, and sublingual glands (Figure 10.1), approximately 600–1000 minor salivary glands located beneath the oral mucosa.

The secretory units (acini) of salivary glands are composed of two types of cells, namely mucous and serous cells. The mucous cells produce thick viscous secretions consisting of mucins and glycoproteins which provide lubrication and serve as a protective coating of oral mucosa. The serous cells produce thin watery secretions which help in cleansing and aid in digestion. Parotid glands produce serous secretions with little mucous content. The submandibular and sublingual glands are mixed, while most minor salivary glands produce purely mucous secretions. Von Ebner's salivary glands, located adjacent to the circumvallate papillae of the tongue, are the only minor salivary glands which produce serous secretions.

Saliva is a dilute solution which is usually hypotonic compared to the serum. Some important features of salivary secretions are summarised in Table 10.1.

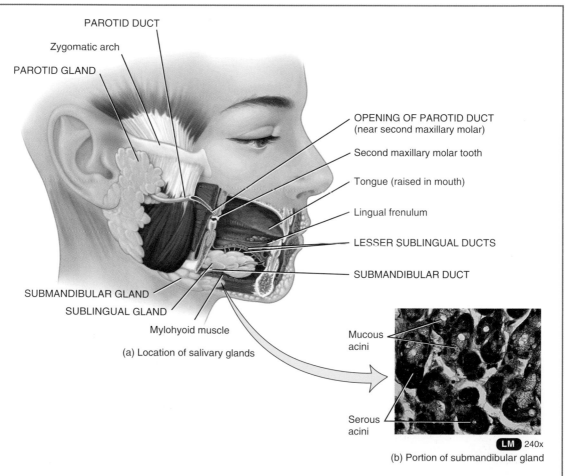

(a) Location of salivary glands

(b) Portion of submandibular gland

Figure 10.1 Major salivary glands include parotid, submandibular, and sublingual glands (a); microscopic structure of the submandibular gland containing serous and mucous acini (b). *Source:* Tortora and Derrickson (2013).

Table 10.1 Characteristics of saliva.		
Characteristic	**Description**	
Total daily secretion	800–1500 ml	
	Submandibular glands	60%
	Parotid glands	25–30%
	Sublingual glands	3–5%
	Minor glands	7–10%
Flow rate – unstimulated saliva	0.3 to 0.4 ml min^{-1}	
	Submandibular glands	60–65%
	Parotid glands	20–25%
	Sublingual glands	3–5%
	Minor glands	5–10%
	Contributes 10–50% of total daily saliva	
Flow rate – stimulated saliva	1.0 to 2.0 ml min^{-1}	
	Parotid glands	70–80%
	Submandibular glands	25–35%
	Sublingual glands	~5%
	Minor glands	~5%
	Contributes 50–90% of total daily saliva	
Ph	6.8–7.4	

Composition

The main constituent of saliva is water (99%). Other constituents include:

• Electrolytes: The main electrolytes in saliva are sodium, potassium, calcium, magnesium, chloride, bicarbonate, phosphate, fluoride, thiocyanate, sulphate, and iodine.
• Proteins: Proteins in the saliva are produced by salivary acini as well as being derived from serum and consist of enzymes and antimicrobial factors.
  ○ Proteins of acinar cell origin include: lipase, amylase, mucous glycoproteins, proline-rich glycoproteins, cystatins, tyrosine-rich proteins (statherin), histidine-rich proteins, and peroxidase.
  ○ Proteins of non-acinar cell origin include lysosome, immunoglobulin A (IgA), epidermal-derived growth factor (EDGF), nerve growth factor, and kallikrein.

The saliva produced by the acini of the salivary glands undergoes some modifications as it passes through the ducts prior to secretion in the oral cavity. The main ductal modifications include active reabsorption of sodium into the plasma and secretion of potassium into the duct lumen. Chloride is also reabsorbed passively, while bicarbonate concentration in the saliva increases as it is actively secreted into the ductal lumen. Stimulated saliva (mainly from the parotid gland) has an even higher concentration of bicarbonate, which enhances it buffering capacity.

After secretion into the oral cavity, desquamated epithelial cells, microorganisms, crevicular fluid, and food remnants are mixed with saliva.

Functions

Saliva performs an important role in the maintenance of oral health.

• *Lubrication:* Mucins and glycoproteins lubricate the oral tissues, which reduces mechanical, thermal, and chemical irritation. Lubrication also helps in mastication, swallowing, and speech. Moreover, lubrication aids in the adaptation to dental prosthesis, such as dentures.
• *Cleansing:* Saliva provides a cleansing action and aids in the clearance of food particles from the oral cavity. The cleansing action also reduces plaque accumulation in the oral cavity.

• *Taste perception:* Saliva acts as a solvent for taste stimuli in food and other ingested substances, such as drugs. The taste stimuli dissolved in saliva are carried to the taste buds to initiate taste perception (gustation).

• *Digestion:* Saliva lubricates the food and aids in the formation of a bolus prior to swallowing. Salivary amylase helps in carbohydrate digestion by breaking down starch into maltose and glucose. Salivary lipase initiates the digestion of fats.

• *Regulation of water balance:* Reduction in salivary flow stimulates the thirst mechanism, which helps in water regulation.

• *Antimicrobial actions:* Saliva contains several antimicrobial factors including:

  ◦ *Glycoproteins, proline-rich proteins, histidine-rich proteins*, and *statherins* agglutinate microorganisms, prevent their adherence to oral tissues, and help their clearance from the oral cavity.

  ◦ *IgA* in saliva has antimicrobial properties.

  ◦ *Lysozyme*, an enzyme, hydrolyses polysaccharides of bacterial cell walls, causing cell lysis.

  ◦ *Lactoferrin*, an iron-binding protein, enhances the antimicrobial actions of antibodies.

  ◦ *Peroxidase* from acinar cells, in the presence of H_2O_2, catalyses the conversion of thiocyanate (formed by ductal cells) into hypothiocyanate, which is bacteriostatic.

• *Buffering:* Bicarbonate ions in the saliva help to maintain the pH of the oral cavity. The bicarbonate concentration of saliva is higher in stimulated saliva, which increases its buffering action and helps to neutralise dietary and plaque acids. Phosphate, urea, and negatively charged residues of salivary proteins also contribute to the buffering actions of saliva.

• *Tooth maturation and remineralisation:* Saliva contributes to post-eruptive tooth maturation by promoting mineral deposition into surface enamel. Moreover, it helps in the remineralisation of enamel before actual cavitation. The acquired enamel pellicle (AEP) formed by salivary proteins concentrates calcium and phosphate against enamel surface and helps in its remineralisation. This process is facilitated by the presence of fluoride ions in the saliva.

It needs to be reiterated that several actions of saliva (cleansing, buffering, antimicrobial, and promotion of enamel remineralisation) play an important role in reducing tooth decay (dental caries).

Regulation of Salivary Secretion

Salivary secretion is stimulated by the thought, aroma, and noise of food preparation. Presence of food in the mouth stimulates both the mechanoreceptors (oral mucosa and periodontal ligament) as well as the taste buds (tongue). The secretion is under the control of autonomic nervous system. Mechanical, thermal, chemical, and gustatory stimuli generate signals in afferent fibres of the trigeminal, facial, and glossopharyngeal nerves. Input from the trigeminal (V CN) and the solitary tracts (VII, IX CN) sends interneurons to the salivary nuclei in the medulla oblongata. Efferent signals to the salivary glands are conducted by the branches of the cranial nerves. The preganglionic fibres to the submandibular ganglion travel via the chorda tympani and lingual nerves and the postganglionic fibres innervate the submandibular and sublingual glands. The preganglionic fibres to the otic ganglion travel in the glossopharyngeal nerve and the postganglionic fibres are distributed to the parotid glands via the auriculotemporal nerve (Figure 10.2). Minor salivary glands are supplied by parasympathetic nerve fibres in the buccal branch of the mandibular nerve, the lingual nerve, and the palatine nerve.

Parasympathetic stimulation increases the secretion of water and electrolytes and thus contributes to the volume of saliva. Sympathetic stimulation does not increase the flow rate but enhances the secretion of enzymes in the saliva.

Salivary secretion is also influenced by input from the higher centres, including the appetite centre of the hypothalamus.

Clinical Relevance

Reduced salivary secretions leads to *xerostomia*, a condition characterised by dryness of mouth. Resting salivary flow rate of $< 0.1\,\text{ml}\,\text{min}^{-1}$ and/or stimulated salivary flow rate of $< 0.5\,\text{ml}\,\text{min}^{-1}$ are indicative of xerostomia. Causes include: Sjogren's syndrome, an autoimmune disease; salivary gland damage by radiation therapy for head and neck cancer; endocrine disturbances, such as diabetes; drugs (antiallergics, anticholinergics, antidepressants, anxiolytics, etc.); and age-related changes.

Depending on its severity, xerostomia may lead to several symptoms, including difficulty in speaking

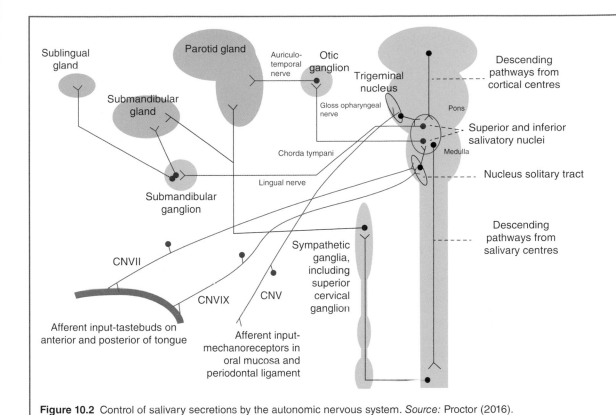

Figure 10.2 Control of salivary secretions by the autonomic nervous system. *Source:* Proctor (2016).

and swallowing, taste disturbances, increased plaque accumulation, and dental caries. Xerostomia also disturbs the microflora in the oral cavity and is a risk factor for opportunistic oral infections, such as *Candidiasis* (oral thrush). Reduced cleansing action and food retention in the mouth may result in bad breath (halitosis). Difficulties may also be experienced in wearing dentures and other dental prosthesis. Finally, xerostomia may lead to a painful, burning sensation on the oral mucosa (dysgeusia).

Increased production of saliva is termed *ptyalism* or *sialorrhoea*. It is much less common than xerostomia and may be associated with local irritation, ill-fitting dentures, infections, poisoning, sexual orgasm, pregnancy, and certain drugs, such as lithium and cholinergic agonists.

Unintentional spillage of saliva from the mouth is termed *drooling* and is usually caused by poor neuromuscular control of orofacial muscles. Conditions associated with drooling include mental retardation, cerebral palsy, Down's syndrome, stroke, Parkinsonism,

and surgical jaw resections. It may lead to macerated sores around the mouth and increases the risk of secondary skin infections.

Gastric Secretion

The stomach produces gastric secretion and its average volume is 1200–1500 ml per day. The pH of gastric secretion ranges from 1.5 to 3.5. Gastric secretion is produced by the following several groups of cells (Figure 10.3):

- *Surface mucous cells* secrete a viscous mucous, which coats the inner lining of the stomach, providing lubrication and protection against damage by gastric acid.
- *Oxyntic* (gastric) glands represent 80% of stomach glands and contain the following cell types:
  - *Peptic (chief)* cells secrete pepsinogen
  - *Parietal (oxyntic) cells* secrete hydrochloric acid and intrinsic factor
  - *Mucous neck cells* secrete mucous

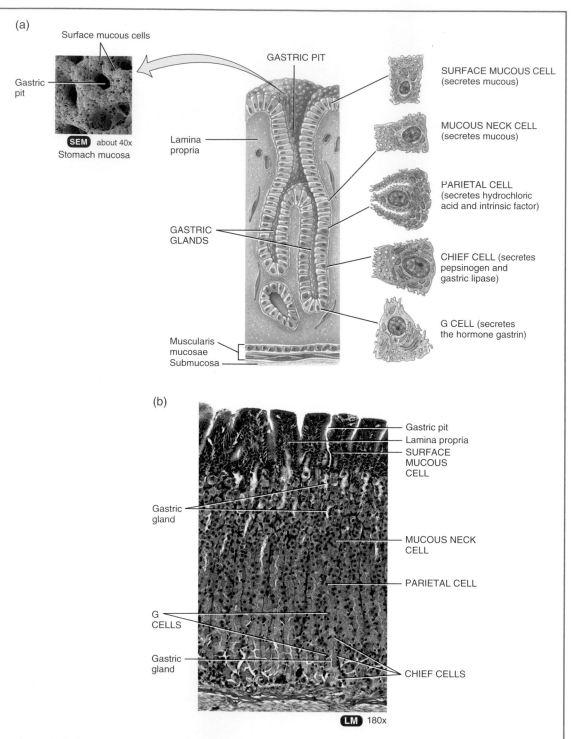

Figure 10.3 Sectional view of the stomach mucosa depicting component cell-types (a); histological structure of the fundic mucosa (b). *Source:* Tortora and Derrickson (2013).

• *Pyloric* glands constitute the remaining 20% of the stomach glands and contain the following cell types:
  ◦ *Mucous cells* secrete mucous
  ◦ *G cells* secrete gastrin.

Functions

The water in gastric secretion helps to liquefy the food, which promotes gastric movements and digestion.

• *Hydrochloric acid* acidifies the gastric contents, which helps to activate pepsinogen into pepsin, neutralise the action of salivary amylase, and kill ingested microorganisms.
• *Pepsinogen* is activated to pepsin by the gastric acid and helps in the initial breakdown of proteins. The optimal pH for pepsin is 1.8–3.5 and is inactivated at a pH of > 5.
• *Intrinsic factor* helps in the absorption of vitamin B12 from the small intestine (ileum).

Production of Gastric Secretion

Gastric secretion involves three stages:

• The *cephalic* phase accounts for about 30% of total gastric secretion. The presence, sight, smell, and taste of food stimulates higher centres in the cerebral cortex and the appetite centres. Neurogenic signals are transmitted via the vagus nerve to the stomach, stimulating gastric secretion prior to the entry of food.
• The *gastric* phase is responsible for about 60% of the total gastric secretion. The presence of food in the stomach stimulates gastric secretions via multiple mechanisms, including vagal reflexes, local enteric reflexes, and release of gastrin.
• The *intestinal* phase accounts for only 10% of gastric secretions. The entry of food in the duodenum stimulates gastrin and leads to continued gastric secretion in small amounts.

Control of Gastric Secretions

Parasympathetic secretion stimulates the secretion of all components of the gastric juice, including hydrochloric acid, pepsinogen, and mucous. Gastrin secreted in response to the presence of protein-containing foods in the stomach stimulates the secretion of hydrochloric acid. A similar effect is produced by histamine.

The passage of food into the small intestine inhibits gastric secretion. This is accomplished through neurogenic reflexes as well as secretion of several intestinal hormones, such as *secretin*, *gastric inhibitory peptide*, *somatostatin*, and *vasoactive intestinal peptide*.

Disorders of Gastric Secretions

Reflux of gastric secretion into the oral cavity may result from gastro-oesophageal reflux disease (GORD), recurrent vomiting, and rumination. The presence of gastric acid in the mouth may lead to erosion of dental tissues, a type of tooth surface loss. Erosion due to gastric acid usually affects the palatal surfaces of teeth. Tooth erosion leads to irreversible loss of tooth structure due to dissolution by the acid. Tooth erosion may also result from consumption of foods with a high acid content, such as citrus fruits and juices, vinegar, and wines.

Autoimmune damage of gastric parietal cells leads to deficiency of intrinsic factor. This in turn leads to impaired absorption of vitamin B12 from the small intestine resulting in the development of pernicious anaemia (see Chapter 14).

Pancreatic Secretion

The exocrine pancreas produces a fluid containing digestive enzymes, bicarbonate ions, and water. The average daily volume of pancreatic secretion is about 1000 ml and its pH ranges from 8.0 to 8.3. The digestive enzymes are produced by the acini, while the bicarbonate ions are secreted by the ductal epithelial cells. The pancreatic secretion is collected by the pancreatic duct which is emptied into the duodenum through the *papilla of Vater* (Figure 10.4).

Functions

The bicarbonate ions involved in pancreatic secretion serve to neutralise the gastric acid and provide an appropriate pH for the action of digestive enzymes in the pancreatic secretion.

The enzymes in the pancreatic secretion include:

• *Proteases: Trypsin* and *chymotrypsin* break down proteins and polypeptides into peptide. *Carboxypeptidase* splits peptides to release individual amino acids.

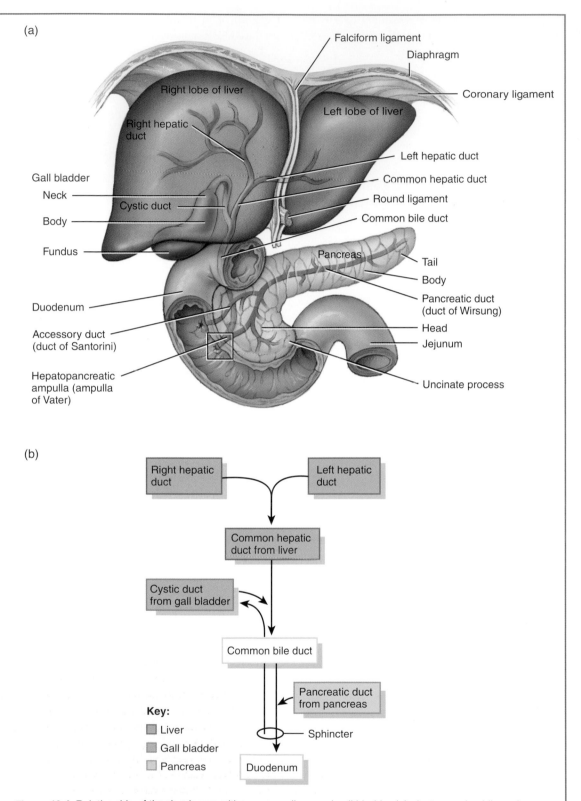

Figure 10.4 Relationship of the duodenum with pancreas, liver, and gall bladder (a); ducts carrying bile and pancreatic juice into the duodenum (b). *Source:* Tortora and Derrickson (2013).

- *Lipases: Pancreatic lipase* hydrolyses neutral fats into fatty acids and monoglycerides, *cholesterol esterase* breaks down cholesterol, and phospholipase breaks down phospholipids into fatty acids.
- *Amylases: Pancreatic amylase* breaks down polysaccharides, such as starches, to release disaccharides.

Regulation

Pancreatic secretions are regulated by parasympathetic stimulation and hormones secreted by the small intestine. Parasympathetic stimulation releases acetylcholine, which stimulates the release of digestive enzymes by pancreatic acini. *Cholecystokinin* secreted by the duodenum and upper jejunum has a similar effect. Finally, *secretin*, produced by the duodenum and upper jejunum, stimulates the release of large amounts of water and bicarbonate ions by the pancreatic ductal epithelium.

Bile

Bile is a greenish-yellow fluid secreted by the hepatocytes in the liver and plays a key role in the digestion of fats. The average daily volume of bile is 600–1000 ml and its pH ranges between 7.0 and 8.0. After secretion by the liver, bile is either emptied directly into the duodenum passing through the hepatic and common ducts or it may be stored for a few hours in the gall bladder.

Composition

Bile consists of water (97%), bile salts, bilirubin, fats (cholesterol, fatty acids, and lecithin), and electrolytes (sodium, potassium, calcium, chloride, and bicarbonate ions). During its storage in the gall bladder, bile is concentrated by absorption of water and electrolytes (except calcium). This raises the concentration of bile salts, bilirubin, and fats 5- to 15-fold in the bile stored in the gall bladder.

Functions

Bile salts reduce the surface tension of the fats, facilitating their breakdown, an action referred to as the *detergent* or *emulsifying function* of bile salts. This breakdown facilitates the action of lipases in the pancreatic juice. Moreover, bile salts form small complexes with digested lipids to facilitate absorption of lipids. These complexes, known as *micelles*, are then transported into the blood through the intestinal mucosa.

Regulation

The presence of fatty foods in the intestine stimulates the release of cholecystokinin, which promotes the emptying of the gall bladder to release the stored bile. Emptying of the gall bladder is also stimulated by acetylcholine. In addition, secretin, like its action on the pancreas, stimulates the release of bicarbonate ions and water in the bile, which further helps to neutralise the gastric acid in the small intestine.

Intestinal Juice

The lining epithelium of the small intestine secretes a pale-yellow fluid with a pH of 7.5–8.0. The daily secretion of intestinal juice is up to 1800 ml. It contains large amounts of alkaline mucous, water, and electrolytes. In addition, the enterocytes covering the villi contain several enzymes which help in completing the digestive process. These include:

- *Intestinal peptidases*, which break down peptides into individual amino acids.
- *Intestinal sucrase*, *maltase*, and *lactase*, etc., which break down respective disaccharides into monosaccharides.
- *Intestinal lipase*, which break down neutral fats into fatty acids and glycerol.

References

Tortora, G.J. and Derrickson, B. (2013). *Principles of Anatomy and Physiology*. Hoboken, NJ: Wiley.

Proctor, G.B. (2016). The physiology of salivary secretion. *Periodontology 2000* 70: 11–25.

Further Reading

Campbell, J. (2018). Gastrointestinal anatomy and physiology. https://www.youtube.com/watch?v=w_54aqc8Des (accessed 1 May 2018).

Hall, J.E. (2015). Chapter 65. In: *Guyton and Hall Textbook of Medical Physiology*, 13e. Elsevier.

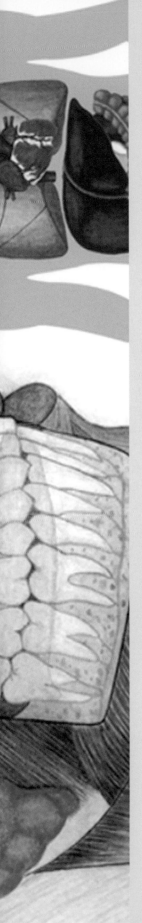

CHAPTER 11

GIT Digestion and Absorption

Elizabeth Prabhakar and Kamran Ali

Key Topics

- Overview of digestion and absorption in the gastrointestinal system
- Common disorders of digestion and absorption

Learning Objectives

To demonstrate an understanding of the:

- Key functions of the small and large intestines
- Digestion and absorption of carbohydrates, proteins, fats, vitamins, and minerals
- Absorption of water
- Common disorders of digestion and absorption and their impact on oral health

Introduction

The complex dietary nutrients such as carbohydrates, proteins, and fats are first hydrolysed into simpler forms by the digestive enzymes prior to absorption by the intestines (Chapter 10). Dietary carbohydrates usually consist of polysaccharides and disaccharides and are hydrolysed into monosaccharides by carbohydrate-digesting enzymes prior to absorption. Similarly, dietary proteins are broken down by proteolytic enzymes into constituent oligopeptides and amino acids. Finally, dietary fats, which mainly consist of triglycerides, are hydrolysed into free fatty acids by fat-digesting enzymes prior to absorption. Vitamins and minerals, on the other hand, are absorbed directly. The intestines are responsible for the absorption of the ingested fluids (1.5 to 2 l) plus the fluids expressed in gastrointestinal (GIT) secretions (approximately 7 l) each day.

Essential Physiology for Dental Students, First Edition. Edited by Kamran Ali and Elizabeth Prabhakar.
© 2019 John Wiley & Sons Ltd. Published 2019 by John Wiley & Sons Ltd.
Companion website: www.wiley.com/go/ali/physiology

Absorption in the Small Intestine

The lining mucosa of the small intestine is folded into small projections known as *villi* (singular: villus) which project 1 mm from the surface and greatly increase the absorptive surface area (Figure 11.1).

The digested carbohydrates, proteins, and short chain fatty acids are absorbed from the epithelial cells (enterocytes) of the small intestine into blood circulation in the following sequence:

Lumen of small intestine → microvilli (brush border) on apical surface of villus → epithelial cell of villus → capillary of villus → hepatic portal vein → liver.

In the case of complex lipids or micelles, the route of absorption is not through capillaries of the villus but via lacteals of the villus and then into the thoracic duct, which empties into the left internal jugular and left subclavian vein:

Lacteal of villus → thoracic duct → left internal jugular vein and left subclavian vein.

Carbohydrates

The transport of glucose and galactose is facilitated by the carrier sodium glucose symporter (SGLT 1). The active transport of each monosaccharide is coupled to the simultaneous transport of Na^+. The process is called *secondary active transport* because the energy necessary for this is not fuelled by adenosine triphosphate (ATP) but from the electrochemical Na^+ gradient which exists across the apical border. The Na^+ gradient is maintained by the Na^+-K^+-ATPase pump found in the basolateral surface of the epithelial cell (like the 'pump' maintaining the resting membrane potential of the nerve cell). The monosaccharides, glucose, and galactose are transported out of basolateral surface by facilitated diffusion via glucose transporters (GLUT 2) into the capillary of the villus and then into the hepatic portal vein and into the liver. Fructose is transported by facilitated diffusion across the apical surface by GLUT 5 and out of the basolateral surface by GLUT 2, into the blood.

GLUT 2 may have a role in osmoregulation by preventing oedema-induced stroke, transient ischaemic attack, or even coma when blood glucose is elevated.

Proteins

The products of protein digestion are free amino acids, dipeptides, and tripeptides, which can be absorbed across the apical border. Because the structure of the amino acids is variable, there are at least four different symporters for *neutral, acidic, basic,* and *imino* amino acids in the cell membrane of the epithelial villus cells. The transport of each type of amino acid is Na^+ dependent, and is analogous to glucose and galactose absorption. Amino acids leave the basolateral surface to enter the bloodstream by facilitated diffusion.

Dipeptides and tripeptides are absorbed from the lumen of the small intestine by the oligopeptide peptide transporter, *PepT1* (not shown in Figure 11.1), present on the apical surface, using H^+ dependent cotransport. The energy for this secondary active transport comes from the H^+ gradient across the apical surface. This gradient is maintained by the Na^+–H^+ exchanger on the same side of the membrane. Once the oligopeptides enter the cytosol of the epithelial cell, they are digested by peptidases into amino acids. The amino acids are transported out of the enterocyte into circulation by facilitated diffusion. It is worth noting that *PepT1* is also capable of transporting drugs such as β-lactam antibiotics, thrombin inhibitors, and angiotensin-converting enzyme (ACE) inhibitors into the intestine.

Lipids and Fatty Acids

Short-chain fatty acids are lipid-soluble and therefore can diffuse across the phospholipid cell membrane on the apical surface easily and leave the basolateral surface of the epithelial cell to enter the bloodstream. On the other hand, disc-shaped micelles containing long-chain fatty acids, monoglycerides, cholesterol, and bile salts which are lipophilic move close to the apical cell membrane to fuse with the phospholipid membrane. Long-chain fatty acids and monoglycerides move out of the micelle and across the apical surface of an enterocyte by simple diffusion. Cholesterol enters the enterocyte by a specific energy-dependent transporter. Once inside the cell, long-chain fatty acids and monoglycerides are resynthesised into triglycerides in the smooth endoplasmic reticulum. Triglycerides then combine with cholesterol and proteins to form *chylomicrons*. The large chylomicron molecules

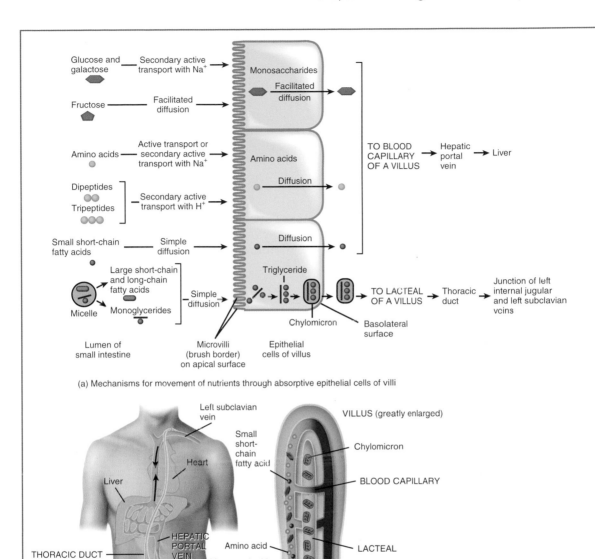

(a) Mechanisms for movement of nutrients through absorptive epithelial cells of villi

(b) Movement of absorbed nutrients into blood and lymph

Figure 11.1 Absorption of digested nutrients in the small intestine. *Source:* Tortora and Derrickson (2013).

cannot diffuse out of the enterocyte on the basolateral side and therefore must be packaged in the Golgi apparatus into secretory vesicles. These vesicles leave by exocytosis into the interstitial fluid and are drained by lacteals of the villus into the lymphatic system.

Following absorption of lipids and fatty acids, bile salts (from micelles) are returned to the hepatocytes in the liver. This recirculation of bile between the intestine and liver is termed *enterohepatic circulation* (Chapter 12).

Vitamins

Many biological reactions require the binding of other molecules called *coenzymes* or *cofactors* to activate enzymes. Complex organic substances, like vitamins, function well as cofactors or coenzymes in our body. Absorption of fat-soluble vitamins A, D, E, and K is similar to other lipids, i.e. through the formation of micelles and chylomicrons which are then transported via lacteals into lymphatic circulation and released into general blood circulation.

Water-soluble vitamins like C, B (B_1, B_2, B_6, and B_{12}), folic acid (B_9), and others are absorbed by cotransport with Na^+ in the small intestine as described above. The absorption of vitamin B_{12} (cobalamin) requires an *intrinsic factor*. Free vitamin B_{12} binds to R proteins in the saliva to form a complex (vitamin B_{12}–R protein) and transported to the duodenum. In the gastrointestinal tract (GIT), the hydrolytic action of the pancreatic proteases breaks the complex into its constituent parts (vitamin B_{12} and R protein). The vitamin B_{12} component is then transferred by a glycoprotein, or *intrinsic factor*, secreted by gastric parietal cells to form a complex (vitamin B_{12}–intrinsic factor). The complex is now resistant to the proteolytic action of pancreatic enzymes and can travel to the ileum to be absorbed by special receptors in the brush border. Twenty per cent of the vitamin B_{12} from the intestine forms a biologically active complex (vitamin B_{12}–transcobalamin, or holotranscobalamin) which enters the bloodstream and gets transported to all cells of the body for DNA methylation and protein synthesis. The remaining 80% of the intestinal vitamin B_{12} enters the enterohepatic circulation bound in another complex called *vitamin B_{12}–haptocorrin*.

Therefore, in the autoimmune disease *pernicious anaemia* (described earlier, the anaemia refers to lower than normal levels of red blood cells, RBCs), there are three different antibodies which can disrupt vitamin B_{12} uptake. One antibody binds to the vitamin B_{12}–intrinsic factor complex, preventing uptake of the vitamin B_{12} and thus prevent DNA synthesis. The second antibody could bind to gastric parietal cells inhibiting the production of the intrinsic factor, and the third type of antibody could bind to the intrinsic factor per se to impair vitamin B_{12} uptake.

Without sufficient amounts of vitamin B12, erythropoiesis (RBC production in bone marrow) becomes abnormal. Cell division of RBCs is affected and the cells become too large to leave the bone marrow. Thus, a low number of RBCs cause impairment of oxygen transport by haemoglobin leading to fatigue. Pernicious anaemia can cause other problems, such as nerve damage; neurological problems, such as memory loss; weak bone formation; or stomach cancer.

Minerals

Iron (Fe²⁺): this mineral is absorbed by active transport across the apical surface of enterocyte as free Fe^{2+} or haem (Fe^{2+} bound to haemoglobin or myoglobin). Free Fe^{2+} is actively absorbed by H^+ dependent cotransport. Inside the enterocyte, haem is broken down into free Fe^{2+} by lysosomal enzymes. Both pools of Fe^{2+} leave the enterocyte on a transporter called *ferroportin*. During circulation, Fe^{2+} binds to β-globulin and is stored in the liver, from where it travels to bone marrow for synthesis of haemoglobin.

Calcium (Ca²⁺): most Ca^{2+} is absorbed in the small intestine by passive transport via paracellular pathways (gaps between enterocytes). Ca^{2+} also enters the apical surface via Ca^{2+} channels. On the basolateral side, active transport of Ca^{2+} into the bloodstream occurs in one of two ways: via a Na^+–Ca^{2+} exchanger (antiport) or Ca^{2+} ATPase protein. Ca^{2+} absorption is regulated by vitamin D_3 (Chapter 19) through formation of vitamin D-dependent Ca^{2+} binding protein (calbindin-D28K) in the enterocytes.

Absorption in the Large Intestine

The main function of the large intestine (colon) is to reabsorb 90% of the 1.5–2% ileal effluent (chyme) which passes the ileocaecal valve (located at the junction ileum of the small intestine and caecum of the large intestine) daily. The colon also reclaims vitamins produced by the action of gut bacteria on indigestible substances found in chyme. Bacteria release vitamins like K, B_1, B_2, B_6, B_{12}, and biotin. Vitamin K is vital for blood clotting, and is exclusively produced by gut bacteria, while the source of other vitamins is the diet.

The colon possesses many long deep grooves called *intestinal glands* or *crypts of Lieberkühn* which invaginate into the mucosa and open into the lumen (Figure 11.2). The crypts are lined by epithelium and consist of two types of cells: (i) absorptive cell with microvilli or brush border, to absorb water, and (ii) numerous mucus-secreting goblet cells. Mucus is a lubricant which protects the epithelium and binds undigested (dehydrated) food matter into faeces. The lamina propria contains leucocytes and isolated lymphoid nodules which extend into the underlying submucosal layer. This layer also contains connective and adipose tissue, blood vessels, and nerves.

Water and Na^+ are absorbed into blood through the epithelial cells of the colon. These colonic cells have specific Na^+ and K^+ (potassium) channels in the apical membrane. Na^+ enters through the apical membrane and leaves via the basolateral membrane into the bloodstream. As Na^+ exits the enterocyte, it simultaneously cotransports K^+ from blood into the enterocyte, which is then secreted into lumen of the intestine, via K^+ channels in the apical membrane. The transport of both ions is increased vastly in the presence of the hormone aldosterone. The effect of the hormone is to stimulate increased synthesis of Na^+ channels followed by a concomitant increase in Na^+ absorption (basolateral surface) and a secondary increase in K^+ secretion (apical surface).

The increased Na^+ absorption from enterocytes at the basolateral membrane lowers the osmotic potential in the cells and results in the movement of water down its concentration gradient from the lumen and into the blood, via osmosis. The route for water absorption is thought to be via *water channels* called *aquaporins* in the colonic epithelial cell membranes, like those in the like those in the epithelial cells of collecting ducts in the kidneys. Water absorption in the colon is tightly linked to Na^+ absorption: the greater the rate of Na^+ absorption, the faster the rate of osmosis.

Because the intestinal fluid volume totals approximately $9 l day^{-1}$, any disruption in water absorption mechanisms would lead to severe dehydration and electrolyte loss, as happens in diarrhoea. This condition can be caused in three ways: (i) decreased surface area for absorption due to infection and inflammation, (ii) osmotic diarrhoea due to the accumulation of the disaccharide lactose (in lactose intolerance which occurs due to a lack of the enzyme

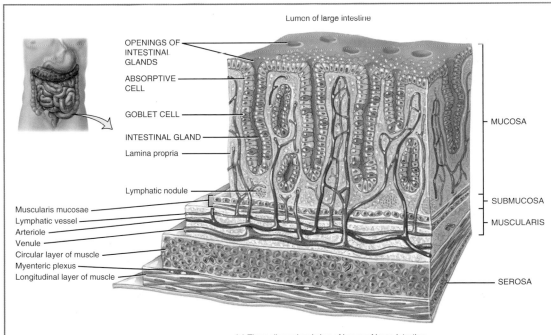

OPENINGS OF INTESTINAL GLANDS

ABSORPTIVE CELL

GOBLET CELL

INTESTINAL GLAND

Lamina propria

Lymphatic nodule

Muscularis mucosae
Lymphatic vessel
Arteriole
Venule
Circular layer of muscle
Myenteric plexus
Longitudinal layer of muscle

Lumen of large intestine

MUCOSA

SUBMUCOSA
MUSCULARIS

SEROSA

(a) Three-dimensional view of layers of large intestine

Figure 11.2

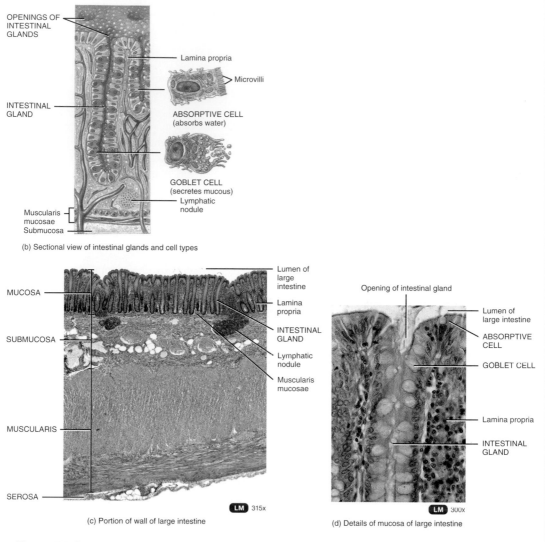

OPENINGS OF
INTESTINAL
GLANDS

Lamina propria

Microvilli

INTESTINAL
GLAND

ABSORPTIVE CELL
(absorbs water)

GOBLET CELL
(secretes mucous)
Lymphatic
nodule

Muscularis
mucosae
Submucosa

(b) Sectional view of intestinal glands and cell types

MUCOSA

SUBMUCOSA

MUSCULARIS

SEROSA

Lumen of
large
intestine

Lamina
propria

INTESTINAL
GLAND

Lymphatic
nodule

Muscularis
mucosae

LM 315x

(c) Portion of wall of large intestine

Opening of intestinal gland

Lumen of
large intestine

ABSORPTIVE
CELL

GOBLET CELL

Lamina propria

INTESTINAL
GLAND

LM 300x

(d) Details of mucosa of large intestine

Figure 11.2 Structure of the large intestine. *Source:* Tortora and Derrickson (2013).

lactase), and (iii) secretory diarrhoea in cholera, as a result of the action of pathogenic cholera bacteria (*Vibrio cholera*), which secrete a toxin. The toxin leads to permanent opening of the Cl^- channel in the apical membrane. This allows excessive Cl^- (which normally enters the enterocyte from blood, via a three-ion symporter for Na^+-K^+-Cl^- cotransport) to be secreted from the enterocyte into the lumen. Loss or secretion of Cl^- via the Cl^- channel is followed by an associated secretion of Na^+ and water through paracellular pathways (space between the enterocytes). Therefore, the excess secretion of fluids and solutes leads to a severe loss of fluid-electrolyte volume.

Clinical Relevance

Coeliac disease is an autoimmune disorder which is triggered by intolerance to gluten, a protein found in grains such as wheat, barley, and rye. It leads to malabsorption, diarrhoea, and growth failure in children. Anaemia due to malabsorption of iron, folic acid, and vitamin B12 is common. Oral ulceration and other oral manifestations of anaemia may be observed (Chapter 14).

Inflammatory bowel disease (IBD) is a group of bowel diseases characterised by inflammation, ulceration, and malabsorption. *Ulcerative colitis* mainly affects the colon and anus, while *Crohn's disease* can affect any part of the GIT, including the intestines and oral cavity. Crohn's disease may be associated with oral ulceration and granulomatous inflammation of oral mucosa, and may impart a *cobblestone* appearance of the buccal oral mucosa.

Steatorrhoea is the presence of excess fats in the faeces owing to an inability to digest fats. It may result from diseases affecting the pancreas (pancreatic insufficiency), gall bladder (stones, obstruction, surgical removal), and malabsorption (coeliac disease, IBD).

Other types of malabsorption include: *lactose intolerance* (deficiency in the enzyme lactase), leading to malabsorption of lactose; *cystinuria* (faulty or absent, Na^+-amino acid transporter), leading to malabsorption of amino acids and specifically renal excretion of cysteine.

Pernicious anaemia may result from autoimmune damage of gastric parietal cells, leading to intrinsic factor deficiency. Impaired absorption of vitamin B12 from the small intestine leads to anaemia with attendant oral complications (Chapter 14).

Reference

Tortora, G.J. and Derrickson, B. (2013). *Principles of Anatomy and Physiology*. Hoboken, NJ: Wiley.

Further Reading

Costanzo, L.S. (2014). *Gastrointestinal Physiology*, 5e, 376. Philadelphia: Saunders Elsevier.

Guyton, A. and Hall, J.E. (2015). Digestion and absorption in the gastrointestinal tract. In: *Guyton and Hall Textbook of Medical Physiology*, 13e. Philadelphia: Elsevier.

Khan Academy (2018). Digesting food. https://www.youtube.com/watch?v=v2V4zMx33Mc (accessed 1 May 2018).

Narayan, R. (2018). Small intestine: Structure, digestion, absorption. https://www.youtube.com/watch?v=0ygBLRNKxEY (accessed 1 May 2018).

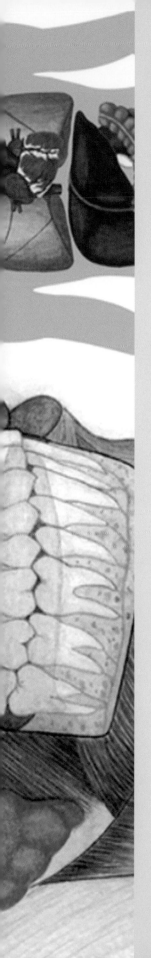

PART VI

Hepato Renal System

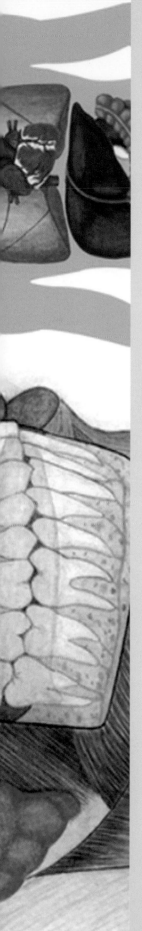

CHAPTER 12
Liver Physiology

Poorna Gunasekera and Kamran Ali

Key Topics

- Overview of the organisation and function of the liver
- Common hepatic disorders

Learning Objectives

To demonstrate an understanding of the:

- Gross and microscopic structure of the liver
- Role of liver in metabolism, bile production, regulation of blood calcium, and erythropoiesis
- Common hepatic disorders and their impact on the provision of oral and dental care

Introduction

The human liver is roughly triangular and is the largest internal organ. It is found wedged under the diaphragm on the right *hypochondrium* (the right upper abdominal region). It not only functions as an accessory organ to the digestive system but also plays an important role in many other metabolic functions of the body. The liver also synthesises almost all plasma proteins, including albumin and the clotting factors. Persons with liver failure develop hypoalbuminaemia (which may lead to oedema due to loss of plasma protein oncotic pressure) and clotting disorders. The liver also converts ammonia, a by-product of protein catabolism, to urea, which is then excreted in the urine.

The liver protects the body from potentially toxic substances that are absorbed from the gastrointestinal tract (GIT). These substances are presented to the liver via the portal circulation, and the liver modifies them in so-called first pass metabolism, ensuring that little or none of the substances make it into the systemic circulation. For example,

Essential Physiology for Dental Students, First Edition. Edited by Kamran Ali and Elizabeth Prabhakar.
© 2019 John Wiley & Sons Ltd. Published 2019 by John Wiley & Sons Ltd.
Companion website: www.wiley.com/go/ali/physiology

bacteria absorbed from the colon are phagocytised by hepatic Kupffer cells and thus never enter the systemic circulation. In another example, liver enzymes modify both endogenous and exogenous toxins to render them water soluble and thus capable of being excreted in either bile or urine. *Phase I reactions*, which are catalysed by cytochrome P-450 enzymes, are followed by *phase II reactions* that conjugate the substances with glucuronide, sulphate, amino acids, or glutathione.

The liver has four lobes covered by peritoneum, though part of the postero-superior surface is placed bare against the overlying diaphragm. The peritoneum anchors the liver to the surrounding structures, including the diaphragm, allowing the two organs to move in synchrony during respiration. Deeper to its peritoneal covering, the liver is covered by a capsule. All blood vessels (other than the hepatic vein), nerves, lymph vessels, and the common hepatic duct enter and leave the liver through an opening in this capsule, the *porta hepatis*.

Blood Supply and Lymphatic Drainage

The liver receives a dual blood supply: the hepatic artery, supplying 20–25% of oxygenated blood, and the portal vein, supplying 75–80% of deoxygenated blood but which is rich in nutrients absorbed from the intestines, as well as hormones secreted by the pancreas (Figure 12.1). The splenic vein also drains into the portal vein.

The liver drains to the inferior vena cava through the hepatic vein. This arrangement ensures that all the digested carbohydrates and proteins absorbed from the intestines are first carried to the liver through the portal vein, before being emptied into the systemic circulation.

The lymph draining the liver is rich in proteins and ultimately drains into the nodes scattered both above and below the diaphragm.

Most substances absorbed from the intestines, including nutrients and therapeutic agents, pass through the liver prior to entering the systemic circulation, an arrangement recognised as the *hepatic first-pass effect*. However, the digestive products of fats, in comparison, are not absorbed into the portal vein but enter blind-ended lymph channels found in the microvilli lining the small intestine (lacteals), which drain to the lymphatic system through the *cysterna chyli*.

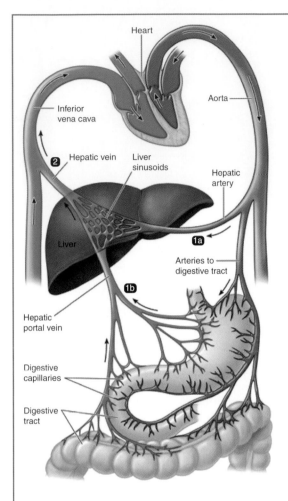

The liver receives blood from two sources:

1a Arterial blood, which provides the liver's O$_2$ supply and carries blood-borne metabolites for hepatic processing, is delivered by the **hepatic artery.**

1b Venous blood draining the digestive tract is carried by the **hepatic portal vein** to the liver for processing and storage of newly absorbed nutrients.

2 Blood leaves the liver via the **hepatic vein.**

Figure 12.1 Dual blood supply of the liver. *Source:* Tortora and Derrickson (2013).

Innervation

The liver is innervated by a dual supply of nerves. Its parenchyma is innervated by the hepatic plexus, containing autonomic fibres, which enter through the *porta hepatis*. The capsule is innervated by branches of the lower intercostal nerves. As the same nerves also supply the parietal peritoneum, a well-localised, sharp pain may result from any disruption to the liver capsule. In contrast, pain arising from the parenchyma is poorly localised and referred to the central epigastrium, in common with other organs originating from the embryonic foregut.

Exocrine Outflow

The exocrine secretions of the liver (the bile) drain to a common hepatic duct that forms by the union of right and left hepatic ducts. The outflow tract of the gall bladder, the cystic duct, unites with the common hepatic duct, giving rise to the common bile duct. The common bile duct then joins the pancreatic duct, which is conveying the exocrine secretions of the pancreas at the *ampulla of Vater* (hepato-pancreatic ampulla). Together, they drain into the postero-medial midpoint of the second part of the duodenum.

Functional Histology

The Hepatocyte

The functional cells of the liver, the hepatocytes, account for up to 80% of its mass. They are polygonal cells with a single large nucleus, though bi-nucleated cells may be found, especially with advancing age. The wide array of endocrine, exocrine, and metabolic functions performed by hepatocytes is evident in their cytoplasm being densely packed with organelles, including numerous mitochondria, lysosomes, peroxisomes, and aggregates of smooth and rough endoplasmic reticula. Further, unlike most other glandular cells, there are multiple stacks of Golgi membranes, with Golgi vesicles being particularly numerous around the bile canaliculi, reflecting their role in protein and lipid metabolism.

The Classic Hepatic Lobule

The multiple functions performed by hepatocytes are further facilitated by the tissue architecture of the liver. This could be illustrated by the *classic lobule*, which best depicts the endocrine and the structural arrangement of the liver. In a polyhedral classic lobule (sometimes described as being hexagonal), the sheets of stacked cells are arranged like the spokes of a bicycle wheel, radiating from a centrally placed branch of the hepatic vein (the central vein). Each corner of the polyhedral lobule contains a *portal space*, traversed by branches of the hepatic artery, portal vein, and bile duct (forming the traditional *portal triad*) in addition to lymphatic vessels. The areas between the radially arranged sheets of hepatocytes (the spokes of the wheel) are taken up by sinusoids filled with mixed blood from the hepatic artery and the portal vein, which is draining towards the central vein of each classic lobule (Figure 12.2).

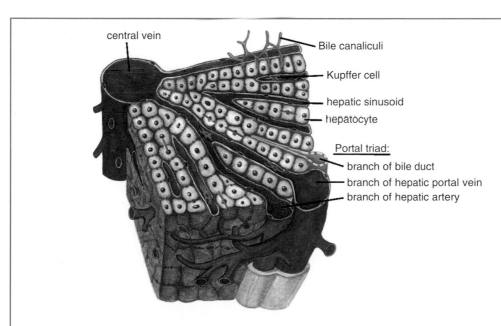

Figure 12.2 Internal structure of the liver showing hepatocytes and sinusoids. *Source:* Courtesy of Melina S.Y. Kam.

Specialised macrophages called *Kupffer cells* line the sinusoids, which help filter the contents of the blood flow, thereby contributing to innate immunity as part of the mononuclear phagocytic system. Because the blood within the sinusoids is moving from the periphery to the centre of each lobule, the sinusoids are described as having a centripetal flow.

The bile canaliculi, which form because of trench-like invaginations on the *apical domains* of adjoining hepatocytes, drain into periportal bile ductules (also known as *canals of Hering* or *cholangioles*), which drain into the bile ducts found within the portal spaces. Similarly, plasma which does not return to the sinusoids from the space of Disse, also drains into the lymphatic vessels in the portal space. Because the bile and lymph therefore flow in an opposite direction to that of the sinusoidal blood, moving from the

centre outwards towards the periphery, the bile and the lymph are described as a centrifugal flow. Hence, the classic hepatic lobule describes an arrangement which facilitates the centripetal flow of blood and the centrifugal flow of the bile and the lymph. As bile is produced by the hepatocytes and secreted into ductules, it constitutes the 'exocrine' output of the liver.

The Portal Lobule

The exocrine function can be understood by considering the *portal lobules*, which are demarcated by straight lines drawn between three adjoining branches of the hepatic vein (found at the centre of three classic lobules), thereby conforming to a triangular shape. In this arrangement, bile would be moving away from the now peripherally placed 'central veins' towards a centrally placed bile duct (Figure 12.3).

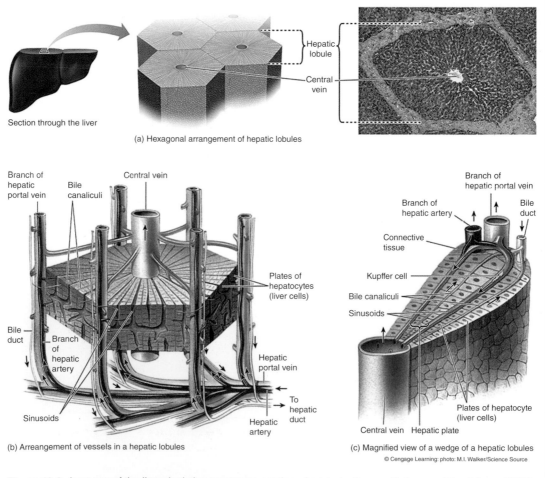

(a) Hexagonal arrangement of hepatic lobules

(b) Arrengement of vessels in a hepatic lobules

(c) Magnified view of a wedge of a hepatic lobules

© Cengage Learning: photo: M.I. Walker/Science Source

Figure 12.3 Anatomy of the liver depicting transverse section of a lobule. *Source:* Tortora and Derrickson (2013).

The Liver Acinus

A further arrangement is described as a *liver acinus*, which is most useful when considering the metabolic functions of the liver. Here, three zones are demarcated, starting with the area closest to a portal space containing hepatic arterial blood and ending in the area draining into a central vein. In this arrangement, cells in zone I, lining the periportal space, are perfused with blood containing the highest concentration of oxygen, while those in zone III, adjacent to the vein, receive blood with the lowest concentration of oxygen. They are joined by an intermediate zone II, thereby describing the gradient of metabolic function, which is dependent upon the supply of oxygen.

Functions of the Liver

Liver is a major site for the metabolism of nutrients and drugs, besides many other functions. The liver is also the main organ of heat production in the body, which is testament to its very high metabolic output. This heat is then carried to the rest of the body through the blood.

Metabolism of Nutrients

• *Carbohydrate metabolism:* Liver helps in the maintenance of blood glucose levels by converting glucose into the storage form of glycogen, at times of relative glucose excess as seen soon after meals (the post-prandial state). During the low-glucose fasting state between meals, the liver breaks down these glycogen stores to release glucose into circulation.
• *Lipid metabolism:* Lipids are transported to the liver from adipose tissue and from the diet. From adipose tissue, lipids are released and transported only in the form of free fatty acids (FFAs). Dietary lipids are transported either as chylomicra or as FFAs. FFAs after entering the liver are mostly esterified to triglycerides. Some are converted to cholesterol, incorporated into phospholipids, or oxidised in the mitochondria into ketone bodies.
• *Protein metabolism:* The liver is the site for synthesis of a variety of proteins, including the production of vital serum proteins, including albumin, fibrinogen, and clotting factors.

Metabolism of Drugs

The liver is also responsible for the biotransformation of many therapeutic agents, rendering some inactive, while potentiating the actions of others.

This role is particularly seen with orally ingested agents that are then absorbed through the intestines. Because the agents have to thus pass through the liver prior to reaching their intended sites of action through general circulation, this is known as *hepatic first-pass metabolism.*

Role in Bilirubin Metabolism

The liver plays an important role in bilirubin metabolism. Bilirubin is a by-product of haemoglobin found within ageing erythrocytes metabolised by the spleen, and reaches the liver through the portal vein (Figure 12.4). As this bilirubin is not water soluble (unconjugated bilirubin), it is bound to transport proteins. In the liver, bilirubin is taken up by the hepatocytes and carried to the endoplasmic reticulum by ligandin, where it is conjugated with glucuronic acid converting it into water-soluble conjugated bilirubin. The conjugated bilirubin is actively pumped into the bile canaliculi to be secreted in the bile (Chapter 10). In the small intestine, bilirubin is converted to urobilinogen by intestinal bacteria that remove the glucuronic acid. While a small portion of this is absorbed back into portal circulation, most of the urobilinogen is excreted with faeces after other bacteria oxidise it to stercobilin, which impart the brownish colour of stools. Urobilinogen is also converted to urobilin in the kidneys and excreted into the urine.

Other Functions

• Bile is a primary exocrine product of the liver and contains bile salts that are essential for the digestion of dietary fats.
• The liver contributes to the immune mechanisms by detoxifying ingested toxins, by filtering harmful substances through facilitating their removal from circulation (for instance via the action of Kupffer cells), and secreting immunoglobulin A (IgA) with bile, which helps protect the intestinal mucosa.
• Initial activation of vitamin D by converting cholecalciferol into 25-hydroxycholecalciferol (Chapter 19).
• The embryonic liver is also the site for haematopoiesis, for a brief period after it is initiated in the yolk sac.

Clinical Relevance

Fatty liver results from a build-up of fats in the liver in obese people but may also be caused by the excessive consumption of alcohol.

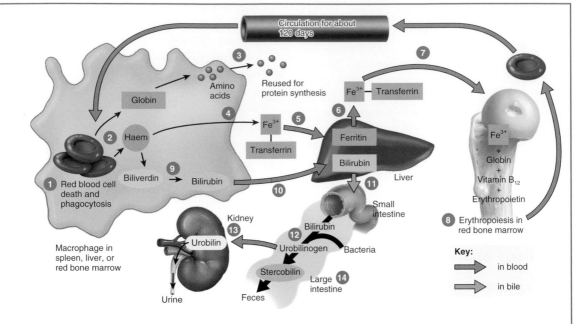

Figure 12.4 Breakdown of haemoglobin and bilirubin metabolism. *Source:* Tortora and Derrickson (2013).

Longstanding fatty liver disease may progress to *cirrhosis* of the liver, which is characterised by scarring and inadequate hepatic function. Cirrhosis may eventually be complicated by liver failure and is potentially fatal.

Hepatitis is inflammation of the liver and may be caused by infections with hepatitis B and C viruses. Long-term complications include liver cirrhosis, liver failure, and liver cancer (hepatocellular carcinoma). All dental professionals must get vaccinated against hepatitis B. A vaccine against hepatitis C is not available at present. Nevertheless, universal cross-infection control procedures must be observed in clinical dental practice and needlestick injuries should be managed appropriately.

An increase in the total bilirubin level in blood above 3 mg dl⁻¹ (normal levels range from 0.2 to 1.2 mg dl⁻¹) leads to *jaundice*. It is characterised by yellowish discolouration of sclera, skin, and mucous membranes. Jaundice is caused by interruptions to the metabolic pathway of bilirubin and is classified as pre-hepatic, intra-hepatic, and post-hepatic, depending on the site of disturbance.

Advanced liver disease may warrant a liver transplant as a life-saving treatment. The liver has an extensive regenerative capacity, with the ability to re-grow to its original size within six to eight weeks, even after 70% of its mass has been excised in extensive hepatectomy. Therefore, liver transplantation may involve 'split organ' transplants, rather than 'whole organ' transplants, with a single liver being split among a paediatric and an adult recipient.

Liver disease may lead to impaired blood coagulation, especially following trauma or surgery. Patients with a history of liver disease who require invasive dental procedures such as a tooth extraction may require a coagulation screen prior to operative intervention.

Many drugs (such as paracetamol) and dental local anaesthetics (such as lignocaine) undergo a significant first pass metabolism in the liver after absorption which reduces the risk of systemic toxicity. Impaired liver function may compromise the degradation of many drugs increasing their risk of toxicity. Therefore, the dose of certain drugs such as dental local anaesthetics and analgesics (such as paracetamol) may need to be reduced in patients with liver disease.

References

Tortora, G.J. and Derrickson, B. (2013). The nervous tissue. In: *Principles of Anatomy and Physiology*. Hoboken, NJ: Wiley.

Further Reading

Dr Najeeb Lectures. (2018). Dr Najeeb Lectures. Available at: https://www.drnajeeblectures.com. Also available on YouTube.

Hall, J.E. (2011). Chapter 70. In: *Guyton and Hall Textbook of Medical Physiology*, 12e. Philadelphia: Elsevier.

Kierszenbaum, A.L. and Tres, L.L. (2016). *Histology and Cell Biology: An Introduction to Pathology*, 4e. Philadelphia: Elsevier.

CHAPTER 13
Renal Physiology

Poorna Gunasekera and Kamran Ali

Key Topics

- Overview, organisation, and functions of the renal system
- Common renal disorders

Learning Objectives

To demonstrate an understanding of the:
- Structure and functions of the kidneys
- Mechanisms involved in urine formation
- Common renal disorders and their impact on the provision of oral and dental care

Introduction

The human kidneys are paired, bean-shaped organs that lie retroperitoncally on either side of the vertebral column, on the upper posterior aspect of the abdominal cavity. Despite their position, the kidneys are able to move in synchrony with the diaphragm during respiration. They are covered with multiple layers of tissue, which provide mechanical protection.

Each kidney has a central concavity which houses the hilum, a vertical slit-like aperture that marks the site of entry and exit of blood vessels, nerves, and lymphatics, as well as the ureters, which carry the renal outflow (urine) to the bladder.

Blood Supply

Each kidney receives its blood supply from the renal artery, which is a branch of the abdominal aorta located immediately below the origin of the superior mesenteric artery.

The large renal veins, which lie anterior to the corresponding arteries, drain into the inferior vena cava.

Essential Physiology for Dental Students, First Edition. Edited by Kamran Ali and Elizabeth Prabhakar.
© 2019 John Wiley & Sons Ltd. Published 2019 by John Wiley & Sons Ltd.
Companion website: www.wiley.com/go/ali/physiology

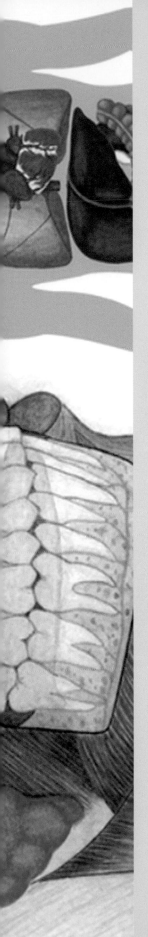

Though each kidney only weighs about 0.005% of the total body weight, together, they receive about 20% of the total cardiac output, emphasising their vital role in maintaining homeostasis. In effect, this results in the total blood volume to course through the renal system, once every five minutes.

Lymphatic Drainage and Innervation

Four or five lymphatic trunks, which are formed by the convergence of vessels originating from lymphatic plexuses within the substance of each kidney, drain into the lateral aortic nodes.

The kidney is innervated by a dense plexus of autonomic nerves which follow the renal artery. They are formed by contributions from the coeliac and aorticorenal ganglia, as well as branches from the lowest thoracic and first lumbar splanchnic nerves and the aortic plexus (Figure 13.1).

Functions of the Kidneys

The kidneys play a vital role in excretion, homeostasis, reabsorption, and endocrine and metabolic processes in the body. They are explained below:

• *Excretion* of water and waste products like urea, uric acid, and ammonia
• *Homeostasis*
  ◦ regulating fluid volume and electrolyte balance through the processes of ultrafiltration and reabsorption
  ◦ maintaining pH of body fluids through secretion of hydrogen and ammonium ions
  ◦ regulation of blood pressure via the renin–angiotensin–aldosterone system (RAAS; see Chapter 17)
• Reabsorption: selectively reabsorbing glucose, sodium, amino acids, calcium, and phosphate from the ultrafiltrate into blood circulation
• Endocrine: producing the hormone erythropoietin to stimulate erythropoiesis (production of erythrocytes (see Chapter 14)
• Metabolic: converting vitamin D to its active metabolite 1,25 dihydroxycholecalciferol, which is vital for calcium metabolism (see Chapter 19).

All these complicated functions and interactions are made possible by the intricate architecture of the kidneys.

Functional Histology

Externally, each kidney is enclosed by the renal capsule. Internally, it is divided into an outer cortex and inner medulla, separated by a distinct corticomedullary junction. The medulla is divided into roughly 12 triangular pyramids separated by renal columns. The medullary pyramid and overlying cortical tissue is called the *renal lobe*. Each lobe consists of a minor calyx which is a receptacle for collecting ducts to empty urine. These minor calices then converge into major calyces, all of which drain into the central renal pelvis, which in turn is continuous with the ureter. Functionally, each cortex is further subdivided into an outer and a juxtamedullary cortex, while each medulla is made up of an outer and an inner medulla (Figure 13.2).

The Glomeruli

The renal arteries branch sequentially, leading to small branches (interlobar arteries) that ascend towards the outer limits of the cortex. Here a series of branches emerge from each interlobular artery, each one of which is destined to become an afferent glomerular arteriole, which plays a key role in supplying blood that is destined to undergo renal filtration, the premier function of each kidney. These afferent glomerular arterioles divide into a series of branches to form the glomerular capillary network, which has a fenestrated endothelial covering permitting about 20% of plasma they contain to 'leak' outside. Each capillary network, also known as a *glomerulus*, converges to drain into an efferent glomerular arteriole, thereby contributing to an arterial portal system (Figure 13.3).

The Glomerular Filtration Rate

This 'renal ultrafiltrate', approximating 20% of the plasma coursing through renal arteries, adds up to approximately 180 l of fluid per day. However, the renal tubular system then selectively reabsorbs around 178.5 l of this ultrafiltrate, leaving about 1.5 l to be drained through the ureters, which collects in the bladder as urine, before being emptied into the external environment through the urethra.

The rate of formation of the ultrafiltrate, measured in millilitres per minute, is known as

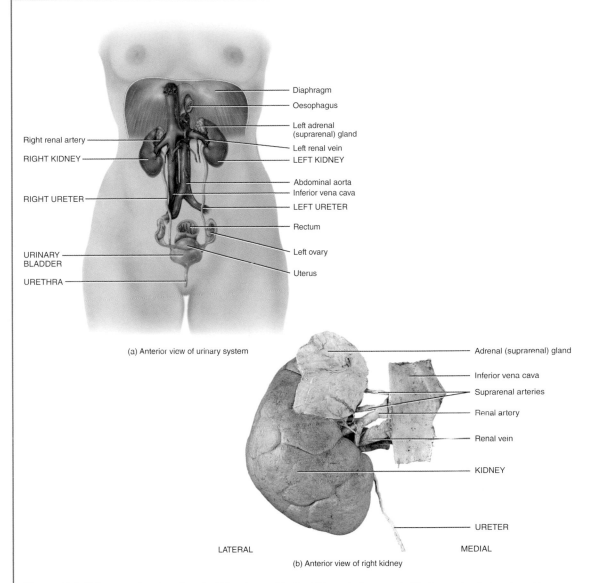

(a) Anterior view of urinary system

Right renal artery

RIGHT KIDNEY

RIGHT URETER

URINARY
BLADDER

URETHRA

Diaphragm
Oesophagus
Left adrenal
(suprarenal) gland
Left renal vein
LEFT KIDNEY
Abdominal aorta
Inferior vena cava
LEFT URETER
Rectum
Left ovary
Uterus

LATERAL

MEDIAL

(b) Anterior view of right kidney

Adrenal (suprarenal) gland
Inferior vena cava
Suprarenal arteries
Renal artery
Renal vein
KIDNEY
URETER

Figure 13.1 Urinary system in a female. Urine formed in the kidneys is transported to the ureter to be stored in the urinary bladder before being excreted through the urethra. *Source:* Tortora and Derrickson (2013).

the *glomerular filtration rate* (GFR), which is affected by a multitude of factors, including the respective pressures within the afferent and efferent arterioles, the blood volume, and the concentration of atrial natriuretic peptide (ANP). The formation of the ultrafiltrate could best be understood by focusing on the micro-anatomy at the glomerular level.

The Bowman's Capsule

The fluid thus escaping from the capillary network is 'captured' by a cup-shaped Bowman's capsule which surrounds each glomerulus. Each Bowman's capsule is made up of two layers: an outer parietal layer and an inner visceral layer that is in close apposition with the endothelial covering of each

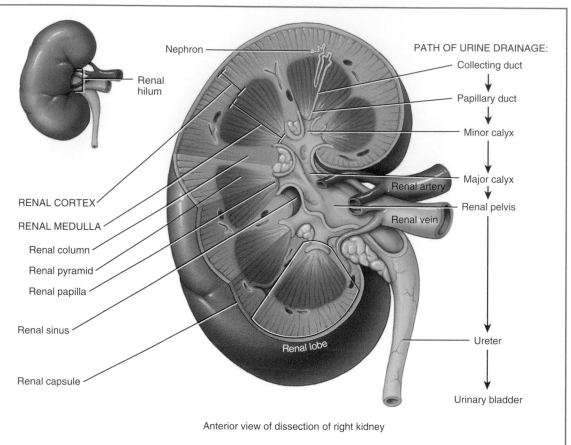

Anterior view of dissection of right kidney

Figure 13.2 Internal structure of the kidneys showing the outer (light) cortex and inner (dark) medulla and associated features. *Source:* Tortora and Derrickson (2013).

glomerulus. This inner visceral layer is made up of cells called *podocytes*, which give off long primary processes that in turn branch off into a series interdigitating (like the interlocking fingers of two clasped hands) *foot processes* or *pedicles* that surround and attach to the outer surface of the glomerular capillaries. Both the podocytes and the fenestrated endothelial cells, which thus lie in close apposition to one another, are covered by an investing layer of basal laminar. Together, these lamellae are known as the *glomerular basement membrane*, which acts as the main functional 'barrier' in defining which electrically charged water-soluble substances are allowed to drain into the renal tubules. Additionally, the slit-like apertures between the interdigitating pedicles, known as *filtration slits*, are covered by membranous tissue, forming a diaphragm which acts as the main

barrier in deciding the size of molecules, such as plasma proteins, that may filter through.

The Plasma Filtrate

Together, this filtration barrier facilitates the movement of molecules of less than 3.5 nm in diameter, favouring positively or neutrally charged molecules to those that are negatively charged. This arrangement ensures that the resulting 'plasma ultrafiltrate' (primary urine) is usually devoid of the most abundant plasma protein, albumin, as it is about 3.6 nm in diameter and anionic. This is vital for preserving the colloid osmotic pressure within plasma. The plasma ultrafiltrate captured by the Bowman's capsule then drains into the renal tubular system (Figure 13.4).

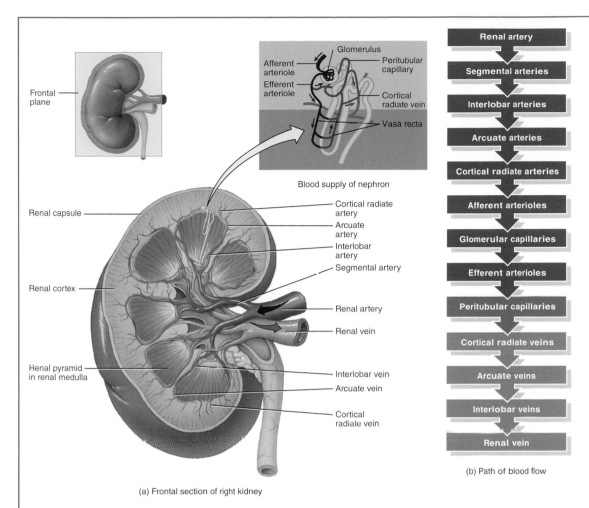

Blood supply of nephron

(a) Frontal section of right kidney

(b) Path of blood flow

Figure 13.3 Renal vascular system showing a highly branched network of blood vessels. The smallest branches of the renal artery are the afferent arteriole and the glomerular capillaries, which supply each kidney with oxygenated blood. The smallest branches of the renal vein, which carry away deoxygenated blood to the heart, are the efferent arteriole and peritubular capillaries. *Source:* Tortora and Derrickson (2013).

The Renal Tubular System

The renal tubular system takes the form of a continuous tube that is either coiled or flat at different parts of its course, lined by a single layer of endothelial cells that vary in thickness, giving rise to thin and thick segments. It could be described as enclosing a lumen that is continuous with the urinary space of the Bowman's capsule at one end, while the opposite end drains into the space lined by a minor calyx.

Conventionally, the part closest to the Bowman's capsule is considered the starting point. Reflecting its

highly coiled shape and the fact that it is a continuation of the double-layered Bowman's capsule (and is therefore near the glomerulus), this part of the tubular system is known as the *proximal convoluted tubule* (PCT). The tubular segment that is immediately next to the PCT is not coiled, and runs a vertical course directed towards the central hilum, before making a hairpin turn and heading back in the direction of the outer cortex. This forms a *loop of Henle*, which is described as having a thin descending limb (directed towards the hilum) and an ascending limb (directed away from the hilum). The ascending limb is further divided into thin and thick segments

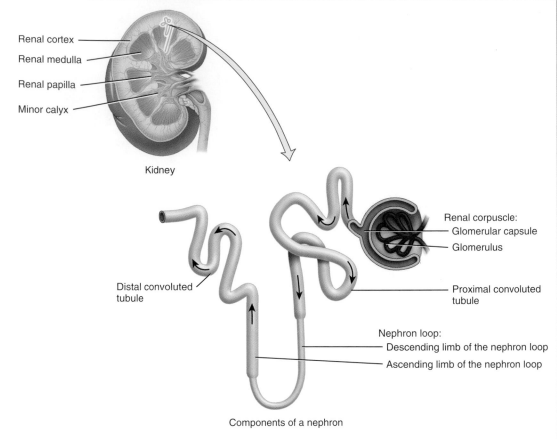

Kidney

Components of a nephron

Figure 13.4 Structure of a nephron, which forms the functional unit of the kidneys. *Source:* Tortora and Derrickson (2013).

sequentially, based on the thickness of the endothelial cells forming the walls of the tubule. The thick part of the ascending limb continues into another highly coiled segment, which again comes into proximity with the glomerulus, thereby earning the name the *distal convoluted tubule* (DCT). The DCT then drains into a collecting duct (of Bellini). Each collecting duct runs towards the central hilum, draining into a minor calyx, at the apex of a renal pyramid. A single collecting duct may receive the outflow of multiple DCTs that open into its lumen.

The renal corpuscles, the PCTs, and the DCTs, as well as the distal part of the thick segment of the ascending limbs, all lie within the renal cortex, while the remaining loops of Henle may either be mainly limited to the cortex or run deep into the medulla before returning to the cortex. The corpuscles that lie within the outer cortex tend to be associated with

relatively shallow loops that only penetrate the outer medulla (cortical nephrons), while those that lie in the juxtamedullary cortex tend to have long loops that penetrate deep into the inner medulla (juxtamedullary nephrons). The peritubular capillary network that arises from the efferent arterioles in the cortical nephrons tend to surround the convoluted segments of their own and adjacent tubules. The vasa recta, which originate from the efferent arterioles of juxtamedullary nephrons, form a capillary network surrounding the descending and ascending limbs of the loops of Henle, as well as the collecting ducts.

Selective Reabsorption

A significant component of the selective reabsorption of the ultrafiltrate occurs during the passage through the PCT, through active and passive transport mechanisms, accounting for approximately 70% of water and molecules, such as sodium, potassium, chloride, and glucose. As both water and its solutes are reabsorbed in equal proportions within the PCT, the osmolality of the filtrate reaching the descending limb of the loop of Henle is said to be *iso-osmolar* with plasma, at approximately 280–95 mOsm kg^{-1}. The thin descending segment of the loop of Henle is also freely permeable to water, but less permeable to its solutes, such as sodium chloride and urea. As the interstitial space within the renal medullar displays a progressively increasing osmolality from its base at the corticomedullary junction towards the apex near the papilla, the fluid within the tubules becomes progressively hypertonic, as water moves out from within the lumen, towards the interstitial space outside, driven by osmotic forces. This movement may result in the concentration of the tubular fluid reaching levels as high as 1200 mOsm kg^{-1} in the tips of the deepest loops of Henle. If such fluid were to empty directly into the lumen of the minor calices, the urine thus formed would have been highly concentrated, carrying with it many important molecules such as serum electrolytes.

This is averted by the unique adaptation whereby the tubes undertake a hairpin bend resulting in the tubular fluid now coursing in the opposite direction, returning towards the renal cortex. The ascending limb, which is the continuation of the tubule from the point of the hairpin turn, is impermeable to water but selectively permeable to solutes, most notably sodium, potassium, and chloride ions. This preferential reuptake of solutes from within the lumen to the interstitial space (without a corresponding movement of water) results in a progressive reduction of the concentration of the tubular fluid, till it may eventually return to a level of iso-osmolality when draining into the DCT at the end of the ascending limb. The selective reabsorption of ions continues in the first part of the DCT, resulting in further dilution of the filtrate, which may drop to a level as low as 100 mOsm kg^{-1}.

However, when required, such as in states of dehydration, the concentration of urine can be increased by further reabsorption of water in the terminal segment of the DCT and the collecting tubule, through a process driven by anti-diuretic hormone (ADH) secreted by the posterior pituitary. The kidneys are thus capable of varying the concentration of urine and thereby the amount of water eliminated, in response to the needs of the body.

The crucial requirement of maintaining the hyperosmolality of the medullary interstitial space, to facilitate the process described above, is met through three complementary mechanisms: (i) the counter-current multiplier system dependent on the differential reabsorption within the tubular loops of Henle, (ii) the counter-current exchange system based on the movement of water and solutes between the tubules and the vasa recta, and (iii) the urea recycling system whereby urea leaves the tubular fluid as it courses through the collecting tubules, but returns to it in the deepest parts of the loops of Henle, thereby effectively remaining trapped within the innermost parts of the medullar, which also exhibits the highest levels of osmolality.

Renal Clearance

The final composition of urine is not merely that which remains after the glomerular ultrafiltrate has undergone selective reabsorption within the renal tubular system. The kidneys may also actively secrete substances directly from the peritubular capillaries into the tubular system. Examples of such substances secreted via active transport and passive diffusion include hydrogen and ammonium (NH_4^+) ions, creatinine, and metabolic by-products of therapeutic agents.

As the ultrafiltrate accounts for about 20% of plasma coursing through the renal arteries, which in turn amounts to about 20% of the total plasma volume, the GFR describing the volume of fluid filtered by the *renal corpuscles* per unit of time, when adjusted to body surface area, may vary between 90 and 120 ml min^{-1} per 1.73 m^{-2}. The *renal clearance* describes the volume of plasma that can be completely 'cleared' of a solute per unit time (conventionally a minute) by the kidneys. The GFR and the renal clearance would be identical if a substance is purely filtered, but not reabsorbed or secreted by the kidneys, providing an ideal tool to measure the GFR. Inulin is an example of such a substance and is still considered a gold standard in the measurement of GFR, despite the availability of simpler, less invasive, approximations (Figure 13.5).

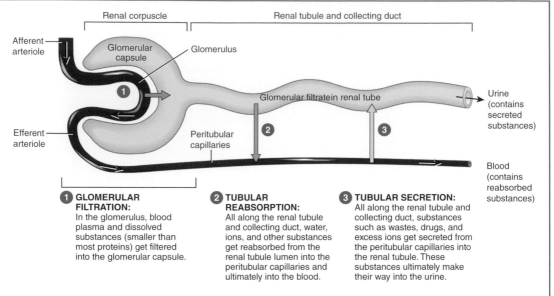

Figure 13.5 Relationship of the nephron structure to three basic functions: glomerular filtration, tubular reabsorption, and tubular secretion. *Source:* Tortora and Derrickson (2013).

Regulation of Acid Base Balance

The blood hydrogen ion (H^+) needs to be regulated tightly (normal value = $40\,nEq\,l^{-1}$) for normal body function. The blood levels of H^+ are expressed on a logarithmic scale using pH units which represent an inverse log of H^+ concentration. The normal pH of arterial blood is 7.4, while that of venous blood and interstitial fluids is 7.35, owing to higher levels of CO_2, which is acidic. Three principal mechanisms are responsible for the regulation of blood H^+ concentration:

- *Chemical acid–base buffer systems in the body fluids:* These include bicarbonate (HCO_3^-), phosphate (PO_4^-), and protein buffer systems which combine with acid or base to prevent any significant change in H^+ concentration.
- *Respiratory system:* The respiratory system controls H^+ concentration by regulating the CO_2 concentration in body fluids by altering the rate of breathing (see Chapter 7).
- *Renal system:* The kidneys control H^+ concentration in the blood by regulating the renal tubular reabsorption of HCO_3^-, and secretion of H^+ in the urine.

Decreased pulmonary ventilation leads to *respiratory acidosis* due to retention CO_2. It may be associated with respiratory obstruction or damage to the respiratory centre in the brain. Conversely, increased ventilation leads to *respiratory alkalosis*. Although much less common, it may be observed when a person ascends to high altitude or be due to hyperventilation associated with anxiety.

Metabolic acidosis may result from all other types of acidosis, apart from those caused by excess CO_2 in the body fluids. It may be observed in renal disease (reduced HCO_3^- absorption or increased H^+ retention), diarrhoea (due to excessive loss of HCO_3^-), or uncontrolled diabetes (excessive production of acetoacetic acid). Other causes include ingestion of acids such as aspirin (acetylsalicylic acid), and methyl alcohol (metabolises to formic acid).

Metabolic alkalosis results from increased HCO_3^- or reduced H^+ in the body fluids. Excessive secretion of H^+ into the urine is associated with the use of renal diuretic drugs, which are used for the treatment of hypertension or excessive aldosterone secretion. Other causes include vomiting of gastric contents and ingestion of alkaline drugs such as sodium bicarbonate.

Clinical Relevance

Chronic kidney disease (CKD) is the well-recognised type of renal disease and results when GFR falls below $60\,mL\,min^{-1}/1.73\,m^{-2}$ for three months or more. Diabetes and hypertension are the most common causes. In the early stages (GFR > 90%), CKD may be asymptomatic. Moderate CKD (GFR < 50%) may lead to anaemia due to reduced erythropoietin production with its attendant oral complications (see Chapter 14). Severe renal disease (GFR < 15%) manifests with lethargy, anorexia, and vomiting. Raised blood urea is associated with platelet dysfunction and the risk of bleeding during oral surgical procedures. Uremic stomatitis may lead to halitosis, gingival bleeding, and painful oral ulceration. The risk of periodontal disease is also increased in patients with CKD.

Renal failure may lead to secondary hyperparathyroidism, which may present with oral manifestations (see Chapter 19). Finally, compromised kidney function may lead to drug toxicity due to reduced renal clearance. Dental professionals need to liaise with medical colleagues to ensure that the drugs administered in dental practice (e.g. local anaesthetics), as well as those prescribed, are safe and appropriate for patients with CKD. Life-saving interventions, such as renal dialysis, are often required in patients with severe renal disease to restore the renal function. Long-term treatment options include a renal transplant, which requires concurrent immunosuppressive therapy to reduce the risk of transplant rejection. Therefore, these patients are at an increased risk of opportunistic infections and delayed wound healing following oral surgical procedures. Some immunosuppressive drugs such as cyclosporine may also lead to gingival enlargement.

Reference

Tortora, G.J. and Derrickson, B. (2013). *Principles of Anatomy and Physiology*. Hoboken, NJ: Wiley.

Further Reading

Dr Najeeb Lectures (2018). Available at: https://www.drnajeeblectures.com/ (accessed 1 May 2018).

Hall, J.E. (2011). Chapters 25–30. In: *Guyton and Hall Textbook of Medical Physiology*, 12e. Philadelphia: Elsevier.

Khan Academy (2018). Meet the kidneys! https://www.youtube.com/watch?v=mcQQGGShmLs&list=PLbKSbFnKYVY2NV3CWR7UR9VLRYkVJVpfG (accessed 1 May 2018).

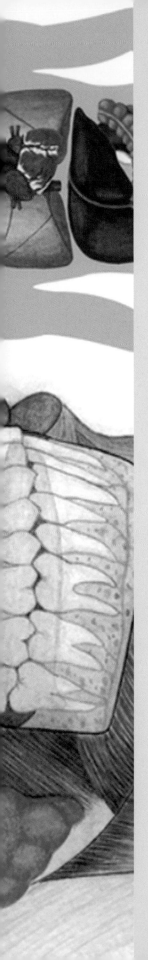

PART VII
Blood

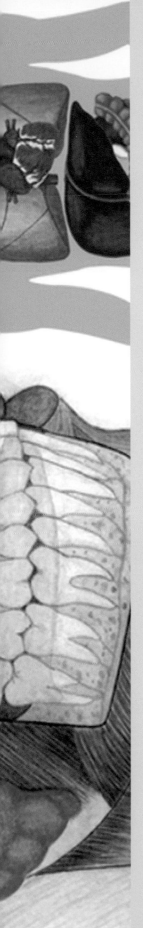

CHAPTER 14

Blood Plasma and Cells

Mahwish Raja and Kamran Ali

Key Topics

- Overview of the blood plasma and cells
- Common disorders of red (erythrocytes) and white (leucocytes) blood cells

Learning Objectives

To demonstrate an understanding of the:

- Composition and functions of plasma
- Production of blood cells (haemopoiesis)
- Structure and functions of erythrocytes and leucocytes
- Normal values of full blood counts
- Common disorders of erythrocytes and leukocytes and their impact on oral health

Composition of Blood

Blood is regarded as a modified connective tissue and consists of a highly fluid ground substance, and mobile cells, but is devoid of fibres. The fluid component of blood is known as *plasma*. It contains water (90%) and many soluble factors dissolved within it, including minerals, gases, proteins, coagulation factors, and hormones. Plasma devoid of coagulation factors is known as *serum*.

The total plasma protein levels range from 6.0 to 8.0 g dl⁻¹. There are three major classes of plasma proteins found in blood:

• *Albumin:* Normal level – 3.5–5.0 g dl⁻¹ (55%). Synthesised by the liver, it plays an invaluable role in maintaining the osmolarity of blood to ensure proper distribution of fluids between blood and body tissues. Also, it binds calcium and helps in the transport of fatty acids, hormones, and drugs.

Essential Physiology for Dental Students, First Edition. Edited by Kamran Ali and Elizabeth Prabhakar.
© 2019 John Wiley & Sons Ltd. Published 2019 by John Wiley & Sons Ltd.
Companion website: www.wiley.com/go/ali/physiology

- *Globulins:* Normal level – 2.6–4.6 g dl⁻¹ (38%). Secreted by plasma cells and play a role in acquired immune response.
- *Fibrinogen:* Normal level – 0.2–0.45 g dl⁻¹ (7%). Synthesised by the liver, it plays a key role in blood coagulation.

The *cellular* component amounts to approximately 45% of normal blood volume (haematocrit) and consist of the following cell types:

- *Red blood cells* (RBCs, erythrocytes): Contribute to between 40 and 44% of blood volume and play a vital role in the transport of oxygen.
- *White blood cells* (WBCs, leukocytes): Amount to between 1 and 3% of blood volume and play a role in the immune response.
- *Platelets* (thrombocytes): Contribute to less than 1% of blood volume and contribute to haemostasis.

Both RBCs and platelets lack a nucleus. The normal range of blood cells along with related parameters are depicted in Table 14.1. The subsequent sections discuss the RBCs. WBCs are discussed in the current chapter and in Chapter 15, while platelets are discussed in Chapter 16.

Production of Blood Cells

All types of blood cells develop from common pluripotential hematopoietic stem cells (HSCs), or haemocytoblasts, in the bone marrow (Figure 14.1). Following division, one daughter cell remains a stem cell of the same type, while the other daughter cell becomes a multipotent stem cell belonging to either the myeloid series or the lymphoid series. Stem cells of the myeloid series produce red blood cells, platelets, and polymorphonuclear leukocytes (PMNs; including neutrophils, eosinophils, basophils, and monocytes), while those committed to the lymphoid series produce lymphocytes.

Red Blood Cells

RBCs are the most abundant blood cells and account for 99.9% of formed elements of blood. The number of RBCs in blood ranges from 4.5 to 6.5 million μl⁻¹ in males and 3.8 to 5.8 million μl⁻¹ in females. Each RBC is a biconcave disc measuring 8 μm in diameter and 2.0 μm (2.5 μm at the thickest point and less than 1 μm at the centre) in thickness. The biconcave shape provides several advantages, including a better surface : volume ratio to improve

Table 14.1 Full blood counts.			
Parameter		Male	Female
Total white blood cells	WBC × 10⁹ l⁻¹	4.00–11.00	4.00–11.00
Differential white blood cells			
Neutrophils	Neu × 10⁹ l⁻¹	2.0–7.5	2.0–7.5
Lymphocytes	Lym × 10⁹ l⁻¹	1.0–4.5	1.0–4.5
Monocytes	Mon × 10⁹ l⁻¹	0.2–0.8	0.2–0.8
Eosinophils	Eos × 10⁹ l⁻¹	0.04–0.40	0.04–0.40
Basophils	Bas × 10⁹ l⁻¹	< 0.1	< 0.1
Red blood cells	RBC × 10¹² l⁻¹	4.5–6.5	3.8–5.8
Haemoglobin	Hb g l⁻¹	135–180	115–160
Mean cell volume	MCV fL	78–100	78–100
Packed cell volume (haematocrit)	PCV l l⁻¹	0.40–0.52	0.37–0.47
Mean cell haemoglobin	MCH pg	27.0–32.0	27.0–32.0
Mean cell haemoglobin concentration	MCHC g l⁻¹	310–370	310–370
Red cell distribution width	RDW	11.5–15.0	11.5–15.0
Platelets	Plt × 10⁹ l⁻¹	150–400	150–400

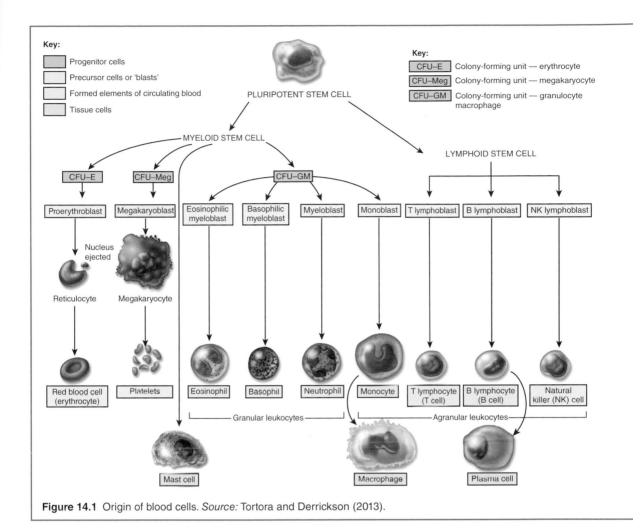

Key:

▨	Progenitor cells
▢	Precursor cells or 'blasts'
▢	Formed elements of circulating blood
▢	Tissue cells

Key:

CFU–E	Colony-forming unit — erythrocyte
CFU–Meg	Colony-forming unit — megakaryocyte
CFU–GM	Colony-forming unit — granulocyte macrophage

PLURIPOTENT STEM CELL

MYELOID STEM CELL

LYMPHOID STEM CELL

CFU–E · CFU–Meg · CFU–GM

Proerythroblast · Megakaryoblast · Eosinophilic myeloblast · Basophilic myeloblast · Myeloblast · Monoblast · T lymphoblast · B lymphoblast · NK lymphoblast

Nucleus ejected

Reticulocyte · Megakaryocyte

Red blood cell (erythrocyte) · Platelets · Eosinophil · Basophil · Neutrophil · Monocyte · T lymphocyte (T cell) · B lymphocyte (B cell) · Natural killer (NK) cell

Granular leukocytes ———— Agranular leukocytes

Mast cell · Macrophage · Plasma cell

Figure 14.1 Origin of blood cells. *Source:* Tortora and Derrickson (2013).

gas exchange and it improves deformability during passage through narrow capillaries. The human heart pumps approximately 3 kg of RBCs per minute. Mature RBCs lack a nucleus, which reduces the load on the heart. However, a lack of nucleus precludes any protein synthesis or repair by the RBCs. Consequently, RBCs have a finite lifespan of approximately 120 days.

During embryonic life, RBCs are initially formed in the yolk sac (three weeks), followed by the liver and spleen (six weeks to seven months). Subsequently, the RBCs are formed in the bone marrow. The main stimulus for erythropoiesis is a low oxygen carrying capacity of blood or hypoxia, as shown in Figure 14.2. Erythropoiesis is facilitated by several growth factors, such as erythropoietin (secreted by the kidney),

thyroxine, and androgens. In addition, nutrients such as iron, folic acid, and vitamin B12 are essential. Other nutrients, such as zinc, amino acids, and vitamins B1, B2, B6, C, and E, also contribute to erythropoiesis. Development of mature RBCs from the stem cells in the bone marrow takes approximately seven days. Regulation of erythropoiesis is depicted in Figure 14.2.

RBCs contain a protein known as *haemoglobin* (Hb), which is responsible for the carriage of oxygen as well as carbon dioxide in the blood. Each Hb molecule is made up of two main components: the *globin* portion, which is consists of four polypeptide chains, while the *haem* portion consists of an iron ion held in a heterocyclic ring known as *porphyrin* consisting of four pyrrole molecules. The Hb

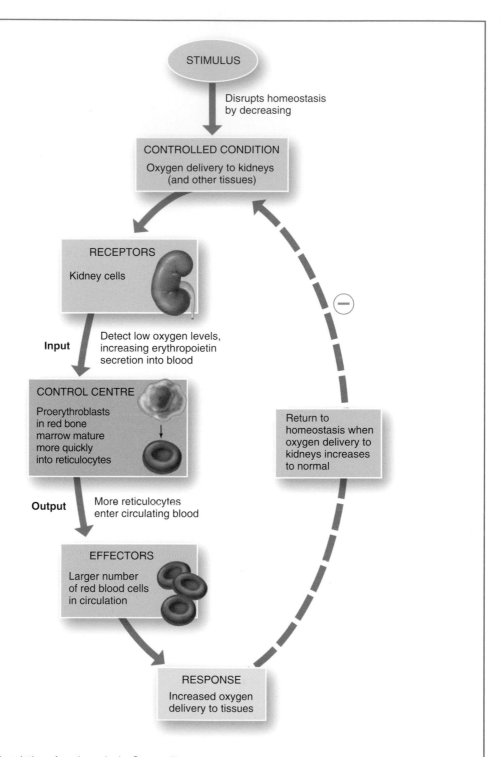

Figure 14.2 Regulation of erythropoiesis. *Source:* Tortora and Derrickson (2013).

protein chains show some variations. Adult Hb is known as *haemoglobin A* and consists of two α and two β chains. During foetal life, the Hb molecule is designated as *haemoglobin F* and is made up of two α chains and two γ chains. It persists until six months after birth, and subsequently the γ chains are gradually replaced by β chains.

Functions

Oxygen transport is the main function of RBCs. Oxygen binds reversibly with iron in the Hb to form oxy-Hb in the pulmonary capillaries. The oxy-Hb is then transported in the arterial blood to the tissues, where oxygen is released and oxy-Hb is converted into deoxygenated Hb. Apart from oxygen, approximately 10% of carbon dioxide is also transported in combination with Hb. The globin portion of the Hb binds carbon dioxide in the tissues to form *carboxyhaemoglobin*, which is transported in the venous blood to the lungs. Finally, erythrocytes contain an enzyme (carbonic anhydrase) which catalyses the conversion of carbon dioxide into water and bicarbonate ions, which is responsible for 85% carbon dioxide transport in the blood. Carbon dioxide is acidic and its conversion into bicarbonate ions prevents a drop in the pH of blood. Therefore, RBCs contribute to the buffer system of the body.

Disorders of Red Blood Cells

Anaemia

Anaemia is the term for a reduced oxygen-carrying capacity of blood and may result from a reduced number of RBCs or reduced Hb. In adults, Hb concentration below $135\,gl^{-1}$ (males) or $115\,gl^{-1}$ (females) indicates anaemia. It is the most common disorder affecting RBCs and can result from either decreased production or increased loss/destruction of RBCs.

Decreased Production

• *Nutritional deficiencies* may be associated with reduced intake, absorption, or availability of iron, folic acid, and vitamin B12.
• *Renal disease* may be associated with decreased production of erythropoietin.

• *Chronic diseases*, such as hypopituitarism, hypothyroidism, hypoadrenocorticism, and of the liver, may be associated with anaemia.
• *Aplastic anaemia* is characterised by the inability of the bone marrow to produce RBCs due to genetic or immunological disorders. Acquired bone marrow damage may be caused by drugs, chemicals, radiation, and infections.
• *Thalassaemia* is caused by an inherited impairment of Hb synthesis and lead to partial or complete failure to synthesise a specific Hb chain.
• *Sideroblastic anaemias* are a group of disorders (inherited, acquired, or idiopathic) in which the body is unable to utilise iron to synthesise Hb despite normal levels of iron.
• *Myelophthisic anaemias* are a group of disorders in which the haematopoietic bone marrow is replaced by fibrosis (myelofibrosis) or tumours.

Increased Loss/Destruction

• *Blood loss* can result in anaemia. Common examples include acute blood loss (trauma or surgery), recurrent (menorrhagia, epistaxis), or persistent (parasitic infection, gastrointestinal bleeding).
• *Haemoglobinopathies* such as sickle cell disease (SCD) and thalassaemia. SCD is a group of genetic disorders that lead to the development of atypical Hb (haemoglobin S). Deoxygenation of the affected RBCs results in their deformation into a sickle, or crescent, shape, resulting in increased viscosity of blood, obstruction of blood flow, and haemolysis.
• *Membrane defects*, such as hereditary spherocytosis and hereditary elliptocytosis, are inherited as autosomal dominant traits. They lead to defects in the structure or quantity of cytoskeletal proteins responsible for maintaining the biconcave shape of RBCs. The affected RBCs have reduced survival and are prone to haemolysis.
• *Enzyme defects* are genetic disorders which may affect RBCs. Glucose-6-phosphate dehydrogenase deficiency (X-linked inheritance) increases the risk of haemolysis, especially following exposure to certain infections and drugs.
• *Autoimmune haemolytic anaemia* results from autoantibody-induced destruction of RBCs.
• *Infections* such as malaria and septicaemia can lead to RBC haemolysis.

- *Hypersplenism* associated with a variety of conditions can lead to increased sequestration of RBCs, WBCs, and platelets.

Although anaemia may be asymptomatic, it is frequently associated with weakness, skin pallor, brittle nails, koilonychia, and cardiorespiratory symptoms (breathlessness, palpitations, and chest pain). Haemolytic anaemias may also be associated with jaundice and splenomegaly.

Anaemias are associated with atrophy of lingual papillae (bald tongue), glossitis, recurrent oral ulcerations, and an increased risk of oral candidiasis, delayed healing of oral wounds, and postoperative wound infections. Administration of general anaesthesia is contraindicated with Hb levels < $100\,g\,l^{-1}$.

Polycythaemia

Polycythaemia (erythrocytosis) is caused by an increased number of RBCs, which results in abnormally high haematocrit and Hb concentration. Primary erythrocytosis, also known as *polycythaemia vera*, is caused by neoplastic proliferation of haematopoietic cells in the bone marrow. Secondary erythrocytosis is associated with increased erythropoietin, which may be caused by disorders of the kidney, liver, or respiratory system. Polycythaemia increases the risk of thrombosis, which may in turn lead to ischaemic heart disease and strokes.

White Blood Cells

WBCs provide the main defence against infectious agents and thus contribute to the immune response of the body. WBCs possess a nucleus which distinguishes them from RBCs and platelets which lack a nucleus. The normal count of WBCs ranges between 4000 and $11\,000\,\mu l^{-1}$ of blood and constitutes 1% of blood volume. The total leukocyte count (TLC) and differential leukocyte count (DLC) are depicted in Table 14.1. However, the WBC count may increase significantly in response to infections (leukocytosis), which can be monitored with blood tests. WBCs consist of five cell types: neutrophils, eosinophils, and basophils possess cytoplasmic granules and are therefore known as *granulocytes*; monocytes and lymphocytes lack cytoplasmic granules, hence they are referred to as

agranulocytes. The key features and functions of WBCs are summarised in Table 14.2.

Role of White Blood Cells in Inflammation

Inflammation is defined as the response of a living tissue to injury. It is the key process that recruits WBCs to the site of an injury or infection. Acute inflammation develops because of three key events:

- increased vascular flow and vasodilation
- increased vascular permeability
- exudation of leukocytes into the extravascular tissues.

These events are responsible for the clinical signs of inflammation including: swelling (tumour), redness (rubor), heat (calor), pain (dolor), and loss of function.

During infection, damaged cells will spill their intracellular contents into the surrounding tissues. These 'danger signals' alert the immune system that damage has taken place. Damaged cells also produce vasoactive molecules, such as histamine and prostaglandins, which cause dilatation of the local blood vessels and increase their permeability, allowing efflux of immune cells into the infected tissues. Locally activated immune cells will release cytokines and chemokines, such as IL-8 (CCL8) and MCP-1, to attract neutrophils and monocytes, respectively.

First, neutrophils are recruited. Activated neutrophils are short lived and produce lytic enzymes (perforin and granzyme) that break down microbial cell walls. They are also phagocytic and clear up damaged host cell and microbial debris. Monocytes, which differentiate into phagocytic macrophages, follow, producing inflammatory cytokines, which further contribute to inflammation.

In the context of dental tissues, if tooth decay remains untreated and extends into the pulp, microorganisms will induce inflammatory changes in the pulp, a condition known as *pulpitis*. It is characterised by hyperaemia and swelling of the pulp tissue, often accompanied by severe dental pain. With time, death of the inflamed pulp (pulp necrosis) may lead to discolouration of the tooth. Further spread of infection into the periradicular dental tissues may follow.

Table 14.2 Characteristics and functions of white blood cells.

Cell	Features	Life span	Main Functions
Neutrophils	Multi-lobed nucleus 10 μm in diameter	8 hours to 3 days	First responders to acute inflammation Phagocytosis Fight bacteria and fungi
Eosinophils	Bi-lobed nucleus 10 μm in diameter	Up to 3 weeks	Phagocytosis of antigen–antibody complexes Modulate allergic reactions Fight parasitic infections
Basophils	Bi-lobed or tri-lobed nucleus 12–15 μm in diameter	Up to 10 days	Release chemical mediators during acute inflammation and allergic reactions
Monocytes	Kidney-shaped nucleus 15–30 μm in diameter	Circulate in the blood for 1–3 days	Migrate into tissues to form macrophages which perform phagocytosis Also transform into osteoclasts
Lymphocytes	Deep-staining eccentric nucleus Small 6–9 μm in diameter Large 12–15 μm in diameter	Few weeks Memory cells (years)	B lymphocytes (plasma cells) produce antibodies and provide humoral arm of acquired immunity T lymphocytes provide the cellular arm of acquired immunity Natural killer (NK) cells fight viruses and tumour cells Involved in graft vs host disease

Disorders of White Blood Cells

Leukocytosis is an increase in the number of WBCs over the upper limit of 11 000 cells/μL of blood. It is usually associated with infections, inflammation, immunological disorders, malignancy, and hereditary disorders. It may involve one or more types of WBCs.

• *Neutrophilia* is abnormally high number of neutrophils. It is usually associated with acute inflammation, bacterial infections, or certain drugs.
• *Eosinophilia* is abnormally high number of eosinophils. It is commonly associated with allergic reactions and parasitic infections.

• *Lymphocytosis* is an abnormally high number of lymphocytes. It is usually associated with viral and protozoal infections.

Leukopenia is a decrease in the number of WBCs below the lower normal limit of 4000 cells per microlitre of blood. Pancytopenia (reduction in all types of blood cells) can be associated with aplastic anaemia, hypersplenism, infections, and cancer. Examples of selective reduction in WBC numbers include:

• *Neutropenia* is an abnormally low number of neutrophils. It is can be hereditary or may be associated with certain infections, such as HIV and tuberculosis; drugs, such as, corticosteroids and anti-cancer agents; and certain cancers.

• *Lymphopenia* is an abnormally low number of lymphocytes. It is commonly associated with certain infections, such as HIV and tuberculosis; drugs, such as corticosteroids and anti-cancer agents; immunological disorders, such as rheumatoid arthritis; and certain cancers.

Leukaemias are cancerous (malignant) disorders of the WBCs, resulting in marked increase in their number and may affect children as well as adults. They may be inherited or caused by environmental agents such as exposure to ionising radiation, cancer chemotherapy, chemicals (such as benzene), and viruses (such as human T cell leukaemia virus). Leukaemias are classified as acute (lymphoblastic/myeloblastic) or chronic (lymphocytic/myeloid) types.

WBCs in leukaemia are immature and dysfunctional. The affected individuals may present with tiredness, lymphadenopathy, recurrent infections, bleeding tendency, and enlargement of liver and spleen (hepatosplenomegaly). Children presenting with persistent, spontaneous gingival bleeding must be investigated with blood tests to rule out leukaemia, as plaque-induced gingival bleeding in children is uncommon. Opportunistic oral infections and lymphadenopathy in the head and neck region may also be seen in leukaemia.

Reference

Tortora, G.J. and Derrickson, B. (2013). *Principles of Anatomy and Physiology*. Hoboken, NJ: Wiley.

Further Reading

Hall, J.E. (2015). Chapters 33 and 34. In: *Guyton and Hall Textbook of Medical Physiology*, 13e. Elsevier.

Majoo, F. (2018). Anatomy and physiology: Blood. https://www.youtube.com/watch?v=55mhfZSENKc (accessed 1 May 2018).

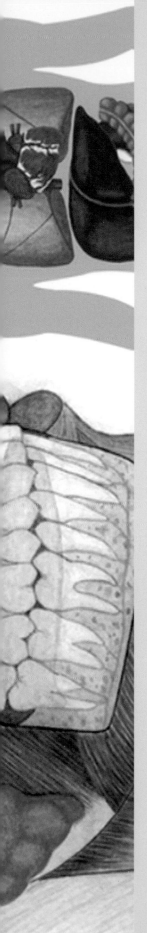

CHAPTER 15
Immune System

Louise Belfield and Kamran Ali

Key Topics

■ Overview of the immune system
■ Common disorders of the immune system

Learning Objectives

To demonstrate an understanding of the:

■ Cellular and humoral components of innate and adaptive immunity
■ Immune response to bacterial, viral, and parasitic infections
■ Common immune disorders, including immunodeficiency, hypersensitivity, auto-immunity, and amyloidosis
■ Impact of immune disorders on the provision of oral and dental care

Introduction

The immune system primarily serves to defend the host against infection by pathogenic microorganisms. The immune system is equipped to recognise invasion by 'foreign' or 'non-self' agents and initiate a protective response. Microbial and other foreign molecules that are capable of inducing an immune response are known as *antigens*. The immune system compromises an *innate* and an *adaptive* arm. The components, organisation, and functions of innate and adaptive immune systems are discussed below.

The Innate Immune System

As the first line of defence against pathogenic attack, the innate immune system is responsible for recognising, processing and presenting antigens, recruiting further immune cells to the site of infection (via the inflammatory response), directing the appropriate adaptive immune response, and disposal of invading microbial cells.

Essential Physiology for Dental Students, First Edition. Edited by Kamran Ali and Elizabeth Prabhakar.
© 2019 John Wiley & Sons Ltd. Published 2019 by John Wiley & Sons Ltd.
Companion website: www.wiley.com/go/ali/physiology

The innate response is *non-specific*, meaning it does not recognise a particular pathogen. Rather, it recognises generic, evolutionarily conserved molecular patterns (usually structures that the pathogen relies on to survive) that any given pathogen will possess. Therefore, the innate immune response only recognises a predetermined range of molecular patterns.

The main components of the innate immune response include:

• *Mechanical barriers:* Epithelial surfaces such as the skin, the lining of the gastrointestinal tract (GIT) and airways of the lungs, all provide mechanical barriers to invasion.
• *Cellular components:* These include professional antigen presenting cells, phagocytes, and granulocytes, along with natural killer cells, that recognise antigens and communicate with the adaptive response (figure 15.1).

• *Humoral components:* The major humoral component of the innate immune response is the complement system. Secreted products such as acid in the stomach, lysozyme in tears and saliva, and sebum also come under this heading.

Antigen Recognition, Processing, and Presentation

Antigen presenting cells (APCs), such as macrophages and dendritic cells, recognise pathogenic microorganisms by a range of receptors displayed at the cell surface, and in the cytoplasm. These receptors are commonly referred to as *pattern recognition receptors* (PRRs). Around a dozen types of PRR recognise different molecular structures. Activation of PRRs will initiate an intracellular signalling cascade carrying information to the nucleus, resulting in transcription of genes involved in host defence. The receptor-bound pathogen is

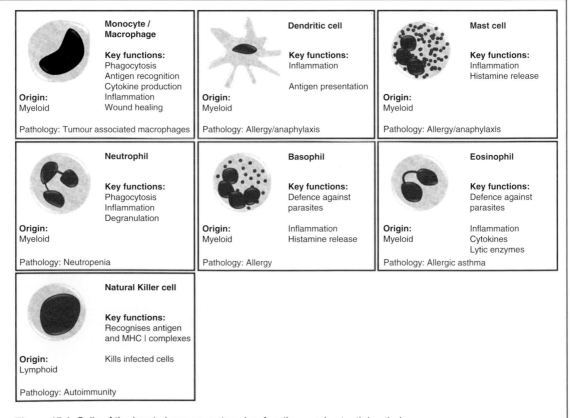

Figure 15.1 Cells of the innate immune system: key functions and potential pathology.

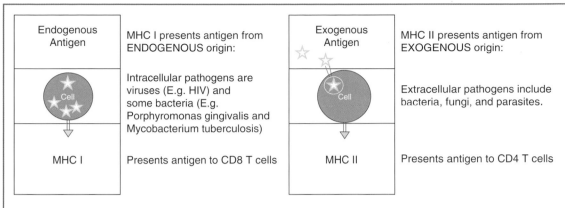

Figure 15.2 Major histocompatibility complex and antigen presentation.

then internalised into a phagosome, which fuses with a lysosome in the cytoplasm, forming a phago-lysosome. Enzymes such as lysozyme break down the pathogen into small antigenic fragments. A fragment of antigen is loaded on to a specialised antigen-presenting molecule (major histocompatibility complex, or MHC) and presented on the cell surface to lymphocytes (Figure 15.2). At the same time, the APC will produce cytokines that direct the appropriate adaptive immune response and recruit additional immune cells to the site of the infection.

Complement

Complement comprises a series of enzymatically active proteins (C1–C9) in the blood that undergo sequential activation (much like that of the clotting cascade). There are three pathways of activation: classical, alternative, and lectin. Regardless of the route of activation, all three pathways converge at point C3 (Figure 15.3). The major end products of complement activation are inflammation and formation of the membrane attack complex (MAC). The MAC inserts itself into the membrane of a microorganism and forms a ring, allowing the contents of the pathogenic cells to spill out into the tissues, causing cell death. The products are mopped up by the phagocytes that were recruited by C3a and C5a. Further outcomes of complement activation include opsonisation of pathogens (see below), regulation of plasma cell antibody production, phagocyte chemo-attraction, and mast cell degranulation.

Clearance of Pathogens and Cell Debris: Opsonisation and Phagocytosis

Macrophages and neutrophils mop up invading pathogens and cell debris. A process called *opsonisation* helps the phagocytes to take up pathogens. Complement fragments and antibodies bind to the surface of a pathogen. This leaves the free end of the complement fragment or antibody exposed. Neutrophils and macrophages recognise the free ends (fragment crystallisable, or Fc, regions; Table 15.1) and bind to them, allowing them to ingest and destroy the microbe. Macrophages, neutrophils, and dendritic cells that have encountered a pathogen signal to the adaptive system for help.

Adaptive immunity

Adaptive immunity provides the second line of defence against pathogens. The *adaptive response* recognises structures *specific* to a particular pathogen, and can provide a targeted response. It is more *diverse* because it is able to recognise any given molecule on any given pathogen. However, it takes several days for an adaptive response to develop, so each pathogen is 'remembered' and the lymphocytes are primed to respond quickly if they encounter the same pathogen in the future.

The adaptive response is dependent on two types of lymphocytes: T cells and B cells (Figure 15.4). Lymphocytes originate in the bone marrow as lymphoid stem cells. Immature T cells leave the bone marrow and migrate to the *thymus* to continue their development into naive T cells (T cells = thymus).

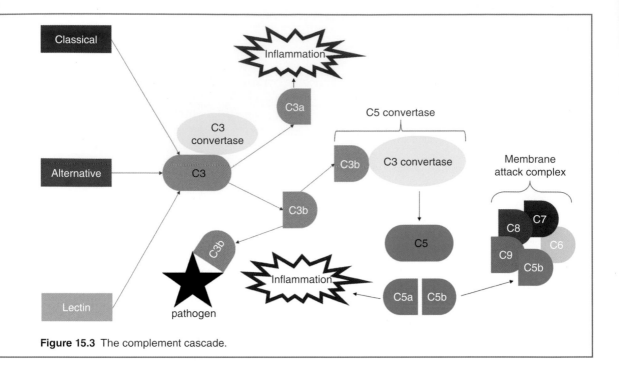

Figure 15.3 The complement cascade.

B cells continue to develop into naive B cells in the bone marrow (B cells = bone marrow). Naive lymphocytes circulate between the bloodstream and lymphoid tissues, looking for antigen. Once they recognise an antigen, they become activated and begin to proliferate. It takes three to five days for lymphocytes to generate enough copies of themselves to fight an infection.

Lymphocytes are equipped with a range of specific characteristics to defend against a particular pathogen. The *cellular* arm of the adaptive immune system comprises T cells and the *humoral* arm is provided by immunoglobulins produced by B cells following their activation into plasma cells. Cell-mediated immunity deals with pathogens that invade the intracellular space (viruses and some bacterial species), while humoral immunity deals with pathogens that invade the extracellular spaces (such as most bacteria, fungi, and parasites).

Subsets of T cells perform distinct immunological functions: type 1 T helper cells (Th1) produce interferon gamma (IFNγ) and activate macrophages to kill ingested microbes. Type 2 T helper cells (Th2) produce IL-4 and IL-5, which help defend against parasites and encourage wound healing. Th17 cells produce IL-17, IL-21, and IL-22, which promote epithelial barrier function and production of antimicrobial peptides at the epithelial surface. They are often implicated in autoimmune reactions. T regulatory cells (Treg) produce IL-10 and TGF-β and promote resolution of inflammation and wound healing. Th2 cells also activate B cells and the antibody response.

Activated B cells (known as *plasma cells*) produce antibodies (immunoglobulin, or Ig). There is a range of Ig isoforms, each with different functions. IgM is the first isoform detectable in a B cell response and is an indicator of early infection. IgM is replaced by IgG as B cells undergo a process of affinity maturation, where the antigen-binding sites of the Ig molecule are refined to become more specific to the invading pathogen (Ig class-switching).

The basic structure of an immunoglobulin is Y-shaped (Figure 15.5). Each Y consists of four polypeptide chains: two light chains and two heavy chains. The chemical and biological differences between the five classes of immunoglobulin

Table 15.1 Immunoglobulin isoforms and functions.

Immunoglobulin isoform	Location	Function	Associated immunopathology
IgA (Alpha)	Mucosal surfaces Saliva	Inhibits binding of microbes to epithelial cells	IgA nephropathy: IgA lacking in galactose is recognised as foreign by other Ig isotypes which bind to the faulty IgA, resulting in the formation of immune complexes. These complexes deposit in the glomeruli and cause inflammation and tissue damage
IgD (Delta)	B cell surface	B cell receptor	
IgE (Epsilon)	Plasma Tissues	Activates mast cells	Allergy/hypersensitivity (see below)
IgG (Gamma)	Plasma Gingival crevicular fluid	Opsonisation, neutralisation	Autoimmunity, e.g. primary Sjogren's syndrome
IgM (Mu)	Plasma B cell surface	Agglutination B cell receptor	X-linked hyper-IgM syndrome Mutations in co-stimulatory molecules (CD40L) expressed on T cells means that B cells cannot undergo Ig class switching and only produce IgM

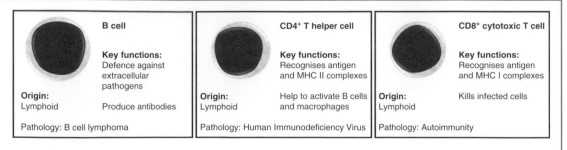

Figure 15.4 Major classes of adaptive immune cells.

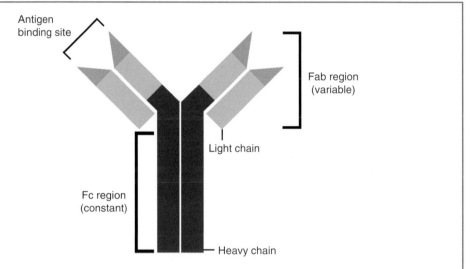

Figure 15.5 Antibody anatomy: the Fc region is highly variable to recognise a (almost) limitless range of antigenic shapes (epitopes). A process called 'somatic hyper-mutation', where genes for antigen binding sites are rearranged, gives rise to millions of possible antigen binding sites. The Fc region is constant; it is recognised by Fc receptors on phagocytes, NK cells, mast cells, basophils and eosinophils, and promotes phagocytosis and degranulation.

are due to differences in their heavy chain structure and whether or not they exist as monomers (IgG, IgD, IgE), dimers (IgA), or pentamers (IgM).

Defence Against Extracellular Bacteria (Humoral Response)

Major Effector Cells: B Cells and CD4⁺ T Helper Cells

When an extracellular pathogen is recognised by an antigen presenting cell (such as a dendritic cell), the APC migrates to the lymphoid tissues and presents the antigen on MHC II molecules to B cells,

and T cells expressing CD4 (which binds to MHC II and stabilises the interaction). Activated lymphocytes migrate to the site of infection; some CD4⁺ T (Th2) cells produce cytokines (IL-4 and IL-5) that help to activate B cells. B cells become activated plasma cells and produce immunoglobulins, which bind to the corresponding antigens on the pathogen, opsonising it and neutralising any toxins it produces. Antibody binding also blocks pathogen/host cell binding sites, inhibiting invasion. Activated Th1 produce IFNγ and tumour necrosis factor (TNF) to induce phagocytes to kill ingested microbes and neutrophil degranulation, respectively.

Defence Against Parasites (Humoral)

Major Effector Cells: B Cells and CD4⁺ T Helper Cells, Eosinophils, Basophils

Parasites are large and cannot be readily phagocytosed. Activated Th2 cells produce IL-4 and IL-13, which active B cells to become plasma cells producing predominantly IgE. IgE coats the parasite; mast cells, basophils, and eosinophils recognise IgE Fc regions (via FcεR) and degranulate to lyse parasite cell membranes.

Defence Against Viruses and Intracellular Bacteria (Cell-mediated)

Major Effector Cells: CD8⁺ Cytotoxic T Cells, Macrophages, NK Cells

Infected cells present viral antigens on MHC I at the cell surface. The MHC I/antigen complex is recognised by CD8⁺ T cells and NK cells. Activated CD8⁺ T cells and NK cells bind to the infected cell and trigger apoptosis via membrane receptor interactions or the release of perforin and granzyme. Th1 cells produce IFNγ that activates macrophages to digest any ingested microbes, and TNF that activates neutrophils to phagocytose debris.

Resolution of Immune Responses

Immune responses are necessary but costly processes. The toxicity of molecules produced during a response to infection can cause collateral damage to the surrounding tissues if left unregulated. Most symptoms and tissue damage seen in an infection are not due to direct effects of the pathogen but are a result of the immune response against it. To limit tissue damage, immune cells have built in regulatory mechanisms that switch off the immune response once the infection is resolved and encourage repair of damaged tissues. Two of the key effectors in this process are macrophages and regulatory T cells. Both will produce anti-inflammatory cytokines (such as IL-10) and growth factors (TGF-β), which will suppress further inflammation and initiate migration of reparatory fibroblasts and deposition of collagen. Failure to regulate immune responses is a key feature of most immunopathologies.

Immunopathology

Hypersensitivity

Type I: Immediate hypersensitivity

IgE antibodies formed in response to an allergen bind to mast cells and basophils through the IgE Fc region, causing them to degranulate. The cells release potent vasodilator histamine, and other molecules such as leukotrienes, thromboxanes, and prostaglandins. Within minutes after exposure, itching, hives, and skin erythema appear followed by bronchospasm, respiratory distress, and hypotension. Individuals with a previous history of allergy to various drugs and dental materials used in dentistry may develop anaphylaxis. It is a potentially fatal medical emergency and requires prompt management.

Type II: Antibody dependant cell-mediated cytotoxicity (ADCC)

Mediated by IgG or IgM inappropriately bound to host cells or extracellular matrix. NK cells recognise the Fc portion of tissue-bound Ig and become activated to produce perforin and granzyme, which destroy the host cells. Ig-dependent activation of the classical complement pathway, resulting in formation of MAC at the cell surface, can also destroy host tissues (autoimmunity). Blood transfusion from an incompatible donor and autoimmune thrombocytopenia are classic examples of type II hypersensitivity.

Type III: Immune complex-mediated hypersensitivity

Mediated by complexes of Ig and antigen circulating in blood. Complexes deposit in blood vessels, attracting neutrophils to clear them. Neutrophils release granules as the complexes are too large to phagocytose, causing damage to the endothelium. Type III hypersensitivity reactions may result from exogenous (e.g. bacterial) as well as endogenous antigens in the host cells.

Type IV: Cell mediated (delayed type) hypersensitivity

Mediated by T cells and monocytes/macrophages. Inappropriately activated CD4⁺ T cells produce inflammatory cytokines, recruit and activate macrophages, and neutrophils, which cause damage to host cells. Inappropriately activated CD8$^+$ T cells target and destroy host tissues. A classic example is the tuberculin reaction which results from intracutaneous injection of tuberculin (a protein-lipopolysaccharide component of the tubercle bacillus) in a previously sensitized individual. It leads to reddening and induration of the site within 8–12 hours, peaks in 24–72 hours, and thereafter slowly subsides. Contact allergy to amalgam restorations resulting in mucositis and oral lichenoid reactions also represents type IV hypersensitivity. Other examples include contact dermatitis, Crohn's disease, and graft-versus-host disease.

Immunodeficiency

Immunodeficiency can be congenital (present at birth) or acquired later in life. Congenital (or primary) immunodeficiency, such as severe combined immunodeficiency (SCID) is life threatening and infants rarely survive beyond three years without isolation in a sterile environment. Loss-of-function mutations in genes encoding interleukins result in underdevelopment of the immune system, and patients usually succumb to infection. Acquired immunodeficiency involves the destruction of immune cells, such as in human immunodeficiency virus (HIV) infection. The HIV virus binds to CD4$^+$ on T cells and infects them. Infected CD4$^+$ T cells are then targeted and destroyed by CD8$^+$ T cells. The lack of T helper cells results in an impaired B cell response.

Dental management of patients with immunodeficiency presents several challenges. These may include an increased risk of opportunistic infections (for e.g. candidiasis), delayed and/or poor response to dental therapy, and impaired healing of oral wounds. Certain types of immunodeficiency disorders, such as HIV and organ transplant patients receiving immunosuppressive drugs, may also be associated with an increased risk of oral cancer.

Autoimmunity

Immunity is a double-edged sword. Although the immune responses protect us from infections, the immune mechanisms can be directed against one's own tissues. This is termed *autoimmunity*. Tolerance to self is primarily induced during the development of the foetus and during very early neonatal life. Interactions of immunologic, genetic, and exoge-

nous factors (e.g. microbes) can bypass the tolerance, thus terminating a previously unresponsive state to autoantigens. Autoimmune tissue injury may be mediated by antibodies or by T-cell-mediated reactions and can involve type II and type III hypersensitivity mechanisms. Classic examples of autoimmune disorders include rheumatoid arthritis (rheumatoid factors), myasthenia gravis (acetylcholine receptor antibodies), Grave's disease (anti-TSH receptor antibodies), pernicious anaemia (antibodies against intrinsic factor), diabetes mellitus (antibodies against ß cells), and systemic lupus erythematosus (deposition of immune complexes).

Damage to skin and oral mucosa can result from autoimmune disorders. *Pemphigus* is characterised by autoantibodies directed against the proteins of desmosomes in the spinous layer leading to separation of cells from the basal cell layer (acantholysis) and intra-epithelial fluid accumulation. This manifests clinically as fluid-filled blisters (vesicles) on the oral mucosa which later rupture to leave painful ulcers. *Benign mucous membrane pemphigoid* is associated with autoantibodies directed against the basement membrane, resulting in separation of the epithelium from the lamina propria and subepithelial fluid accumulation. This leads to larger blisters (bullae) which rupture to leave large painful ulcers and subsequent scarring. *Sjogren's syndrome*, another autoimmune disorder, leads to damage to the salivary and lacrimal glands from autoantibodies and cytotoxic T cells. It results in xerostomia (dry mouth) and xerophthalmia (dry eyes) with its attendant complications (see Section 10.2.3.1).

Amyloidosis

Amyloidosis is a group of diseases that share the extracellular deposition of pathologic proteinaceous substance (amyloid) between cells in various tissues and organs of the body. Although poorly understood, amyloidosis probably results from quantitative or qualitative changes in the precursor proteins (such as immunoglobulin light chains and acute phase proteins associated with inflammation), coupled with defective or deficient proteolysis. Amyloidosis may be localised or generalised and may result in organ enlargement and dysfunction. Common organs affected by amyloidosis include kidneys, spleen, liver, GIT, and heart. Amyloidosis may also lead to tongue enlargement (macroglossia).

Further Reading

Abbas, A., Lichtman, A.H., and Shiv, P. (2015). Basic immunology. In: *Functions and Disorders of the Immune System*, 5e. Elsevier.

Helbert, M. (2006). *Flesh and Bones of Immunology*. Edinburgh: Mosby Elsevier.

The British Society of Immunology (2018). BiteSized Immunolog. https://www.immunology.org/public-information/bitesized-immunology (accessed 1 May 2018).

The Khan Academy (2018). Human biology: Immunology. https://www.khanacademy.org/science/biology/human-biology#immunology (accessed 1 May 2018).

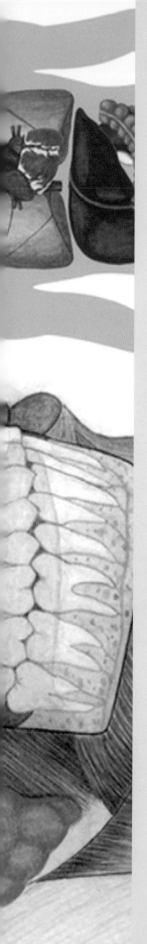

CHAPTER 16
Haemostasis

Kamran Ali

Key Topics

- Overview of the blood coagulation system
- Common disorders of bleeding and coagulation

Learning Objectives

To demonstrate an understanding of the:
- Role of platelets in platelet plug formation (primary haemostasis)
- Extrinsic, intrinsic, and common pathways of blood coagulation (secondary haemostasis)
- Fibrinolysis (tertiary haemostasis)
- Interpretation of common blood tests to identify bleeding and clotting disorders
- Congenital, acquired, and medication-related defects of platelets and coagulation disorders and implications for oral surgical care

Introduction

Haemostasis is the arrest of bleeding and involves an interplay between blood vessels, platelets, and coagulation factors (Table 16.1) in the plasma. Under normal circumstances, the anticoagulant factors in the blood predominate and ensure the smooth flow of blood. An intact blood vessel wall (endothelium) promotes the normal flow of blood, prevents stasis of platelets, and maintains the patency of the vessel. This is achieved by the smoothness of the endothelium; production of nitric oxide, prostacyclin, and endothelial ADP-ase by the blood vessels; and the presence of endogenous anticoagulants in the blood.

Essential Physiology for Dental Students, First Edition. Edited by Kamran Ali and Elizabeth Prabhakar.
© 2019 John Wiley & Sons Ltd. Published 2019 by John Wiley & Sons Ltd.
Companion website: www.wiley.com/go/ali/physiology

Table 16.1 Coagulation factors.

Factor number	Descriptive name	Function	Genetic disorder(s)
I	Fibrinogen	Polymerises to form the blood clot	Afibrinogenaemia Hypofibrinogenaemia Hyperfibrinogenaemia
II	Prothrombin	Activates factors I, V, VII, VIII, XI, XIII	Dysprothrombinaemia Hypoprothrombinaemia
III	Tissue factor	Initiates the extrinsic pathway Cofactor for factor X activation	
IV	Calcium	Facilitates binding of clotting factors to phospholipids	Deficiency does not affect coagulation as respiratory arrest may occur prior to bleeding
V	Labile factor	Cofactor for activation of prothrombin to thrombin	Parahaemophilia (factor V Leiden mutation)
VI	Unassigned	Old name of factor Va	
VII	Proconvertin	Activates factors IX, X Activates extrinsic pathway with tissue factor	Deficiency leads to bleeding diathesis and haemorrhages
VIII	Antihaemophilic factor	Cofactor in the activation of factor X	Haemophilia A
IX	Christmas factor	Activates factor IX	Haemophilia B or Christmas disease
X	Stuart–Power factor	Cleaves prothrombin to thrombin	Deficiency leads to bleeding diathesis and haemorrhages
XI	Plasma thromboplastin antecedent	Activates factor IX	Haemorrhage after surgery or trauma
XII	Hageman (contact) factor	Activates factor XI and prekallikrein	Deficiency may lead to thrombosis due to inactivation of fibrinolysis
XIII	Fibrin-stabilising factor	Polymerises fibrin and stabilises blood clot	Bleeding diathesis
	Prekallikrein (Fletcher factor)	Cofactor for the activation of kallikrein and factor XII	
	High-molecular-weight kininogen (HMWK, aka Fitzgerald factor)	Cleaves kininogen releasing bradykinin	
	Von Willebrand factor (vWF)	Platelet adhesion	von Willebrand disease
	Antithrombin III	Anticoagulant Inhibits factor II, X	Deficiency of anticoagulant factors promotes procoagulant tendency and increases risk of venous thromboembolism
	Heparin cofactor	Anticoagulant Inhibits factor II	
	Protein C	Anticoagulant Inhibits factors V, VIII	
	Protein S	Anticoagulant Cofactor for protein C	
	Plasminogen	Lyses fibrin	

Following injury to the blood vessels, a series of events leads to the formation of a blood clot. A simplified sequence of events can be described as:

• *Primary haemostasis:* Blood vessel wall constriction and formation of a platelet plug.
• *Secondary haemostasis:* Activation of coagulation cascade resulting in the deposition and stabilisation of fibrin.
• *Tertiary haemostasis:* Fibrinolysis resulting in dissolution of fibrin.

Platelets

Features

Platelets or thrombocytes lack a nucleus and are membrane-bound, cell fragments of megakaryocytes (Chapter 14). Their production is regulated by a hormone, thrombopoietin, which is produced by the liver and kidneys. Platelets are discoid-shaped cells that resemble a biconvex lens and measure $2.5\,\mu m$ in diameter (lens-shaped). The normal platelet count is $150\,000–450\,000\,\mu l^{-1}$ of blood and they have a lifespan of 8–10 days.

Functions

The main function of the platelets is to aid haemostasis. First, they help in the formation of a haemostatic (platelet) plug. Second, the phospholipid membrane of platelets activates the coagulation cascade. The formation of a blood clot not only arrests bleeding but also contributes to the initial stages of wound healing. Hyperactivity of platelets also contributes to several pathological conditions, such as thromboembolism and cardiovascular disease.

Disorders

Thrombocytopenia is low platelet count. It may be caused by decreased production of platelets due to bone marrow damage (e.g. aplastic anaemia, leukaemia, and myelofibrosis) or increased destruction (e.g. autoimmune thrombocytopenic purpura, transfusion of stored blood, and spleen enlargement). Functional disorders of platelets may occur despite normal counts and may be inherited or acquired. Von Willebrand's disease is inherited as an autosomal dominant trait and leads to defective von Willebrand fraction of factor VIII, which is required for platelet adhesion and plug formation. Acquired disorders which cause impairment of platelet function include liver disease and renal disease (uraemia). Moreover, drugs with antiplatelet activity are frequently prescribed to patients with cardiovascular disease as blood thinners. Examples of such drugs include aspirin, dipyridamole, clopidogrel, ticagrelor, and prasugrel.

Thrombocytopenia can lead to bleeding from skin and mucosa. Manifestations include epistaxis, purpura (red or purple spots due to subcutaneous bleeding), petechiae (pin point haemorrhagic spots), and gingival bleeding. Patients with platelet counts below $50\,000\,\mu l^{-1}$ may experience excessive bleeding during oral surgery. Moreover, patients on antiplatelet drugs require additional haemostatic measure to control bleeding during oral surgery.

Thrombocytosis is increased platelet count. It is regarded as primary when caused by cancer of the bone marrow. Secondary types may develop due to inflammation, infection, haemorrhage, hyposplenism, and steroid medications. A high platelet count may increase the risk of thrombosis and cardiovascular disease.

Formation of Platelet Plug

Damaged endothelium expresses von Willebrand factor (vWF) which facilitates the *adhesion* of the platelets to the subendothelium by binding to platelet glycoprotein (GPIb). Once anchored to the vessel wall, the platelets undergo *activation*, releasing a variety of mediators stored in the cytoplasmic granules including adenosine diphosphate (ADP). A variety of biochemical changes accompany platelet activation including the mobilisation of intracellular calcium from platelet cytoskeleton. Intracellular calcium acts as the second messenger that drives cytoskeletal changes in platelets and causes degranulation. It activates of several events in the platelets including release of kinases necessary for morphologic change; the presentation of the procoagulant phospholipid surface; the secretion of platelet granular content (fibrinogen, fibronectin, and vWF); the activation of glycoproteins; and the activation of phospholipase A_2. Phospholipase catalyses arachidonic acid metabolism, producing thromboxane A_2 (TXA_2) via the cyclooxygenase pathway. TXA_2 is a powerful mediator of platelet aggregation.

Aggregation of platelets occurs through activation of the fibrinogen receptor (glycoproteins IIb and IIIa) expressed on platelet cells. This facilitates binding of fibrinogen and linkage of the activated platelets through fibrinogen bridges, forming a platelet plug.

Activation of the Coagulation Cascade

The coagulation cascade can be triggered by two separate pathways, as illustrated in Figure 16.1, and involves a series of reactions to convert pro factors into activated factors. The *extrinsic pathway* is triggered immediately after injury to blood vessels, which releases tissue factor from the vessel wall, which, in turn, activates factor VII. The *intrinsic pathway* is initiated by the formation of a complex of factor XII, high-molecular-weight kininogen (HMWK), and prekallikrein on the surface of collagen. Both pathways ultimately lead to the activation of factor X

to trigger the *common pathway*. The activated factor X then catalyses the activation of prothrombin, which in turn activates thrombin. Finally, thrombin acts on fibrinogen to convert it to fibrin.

Fibrinolysis

As repair proceeds, the clot gradually dissolves (fibrinolysis). Thrombin (activated by the common pathway) and the tissue plasminogen activator (released by the damaged tissue) activate the proenzyme plasminogen. The activation of plasminogen converts it into plasmin, which digests the fibrin strands, releasing fibrin degradation products (FDPs). A variety of blood tests are available to assess haemostatic function and are summarised in Table 16.2.

Coagulation Disorders

Genetic Disorders

Haemophilia is a rare, yet well-recognised, genetic coagulation disorder which is transmitted as an X-linked recessive trait. Males have XY chromosomes

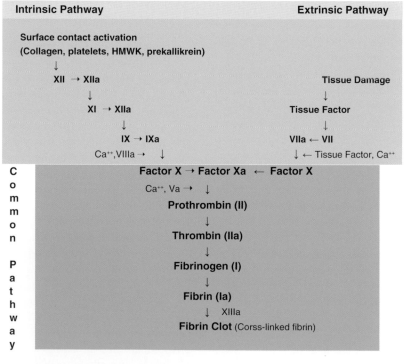

Figure 16.1 The coagulation cascade.

Table 16.2 Blood coagulation tests.

Test	Description	Normal values	Interpretation
Bleeding time (BT)	Time interval between oozing of blood to arrest of bleeding Measures platelet function *in vivo*	2–9 min	Prolonged in platelet deficiency Von Willebrand disease
Prothrombin time (PT)	Time taken by the citrated platelet-poor plasma to form a clot in the presence of concentration of calcium and tissue thromboplastin Reflects the integrity of the extrinsic and common coagulation pathways	10–15 sec	Prolonged in liver disease Deficiencies factor VII and vitamin K Warfarin therapy
International normalised ratio (INR)	Standardises the PT results across different laboratories as thromboplastin test reagents differ in sensitivity	0.8–1.2	As for PT above
Activated partial thromboplastin time (aPTT)	Time required for clot formation when plasma is mixed with phospholipid, calcium, and a contact activator (e.g. Celite®, kaolin, silica) reflects the integrity of the extrinsic and common coagulation pathways	20–36 sec	Prolonged in deficiencies of clotting factors except factor VII Most sensitive to factor VIII and IX deficiencies
Thrombin time (TT)	Time required for thrombin to convert fibrinogen to fibrin Performed by adding thrombin to plasm	9–13 sec	Prolonged in fibrinogen deficiency (hypofibrinogenemia), defective fibrinogen (dysfibrinogenemia), liver disease, and Heparin therapy
Clotting factors assay	Measurement of plasma levels of individual clotting factors		Identify individual or combined clotting factor deficiencies

and can inherit an X chromosome carrying haemophilia from their mother. It also means that fathers cannot pass haemophilia on to their sons. Females have two X chromosomes, and if they inherit the haemophilia gene from their mother, they will only be carriers of haemophilia as they are likely to inherit a healthy X chromosome from their father. Haemophilia in females is rare. About one-third of cases are caused by spontaneous genetic mutations. The incidence of haemophilia is approximately 1 in 5000 births.

Haemophilia is characterised by a deficiency or defective factor VIII and results in severe and prolonged bleeding, depending on the severity of the factor VIII deficiency. Haemophilia is graded as mild (5–50% of factor VIII), moderate (1–5% of factor VIII), and severe (< 1% of factor VIII). Approximately, 50% of affected individuals have a severe form of

haemophilia. Apart from severe external bleeding following trauma, haemophiliacs may experience internal bleeding in the joints, muscles, abdomen, and cranium, the latter being potentially fatal. Haemophilia is managed by the replacement of factor VIII and all haemophiliacs need to be registered. Invasive dental surgical procedures, including tooth extractions, are done in a hospital setting under the joint care of a haematologist and an oral surgeon. Depending on the severity of haemophilia and the nature of the surgical procedure, appropriate factor VIII replacement must be provided.

Christmas Disease

It is also known as *haemophilia B* and is caused by a genetic deficiency of factor IX. Like haemophilia A, it is transmitted as an X-linked recessive trait and its incidence is approximately 1 in 30 000 births. Like haemophilia A, it usually affects males, and the clinical presentation is also similar. Management requires factor IX replacement.

Acquired Disorders

Vitamin K Deficiency

Vitamin K is fat soluble and helps in the synthesis of several clotting factors, including factors II, VII, IX, and X and proteins C and S. A deficiency state may result from malabsorption (cholestatic jaundice), an impaired endogenous synthesis (broad spectrum antibiotic use), and impaired utilisation (liver disease, oral anticoagulant drugs). It may be lead to a bleeding tendency and present with bruising and bleeding from internal organs.

Liver Disease

Liver is the site of the synthesis of blood-clotting factors. Hepatocytes are involved in the synthesis of fibrinogen, prothrombin, factors V, VII, IX, X, XI, and XII, as well as proteins C and S, and antithrombin, whereas liver sinusoidal endothelial cells produce factor VIII and vWF. Liver disease, such as hepatitis and liver cirrhosis, increases the risk of bleeding. Dental surgery in patients with liver disease requires preoperative liver function tests (LFTs) and liaising with the patient's medical practitioner.

Disseminated Intravascular Coagulation

Disseminated intravascular coagulation (DIC) develops as a complication of several conditions, including sepsis (infection with gram-negative bacteria), blood transfusion reactions, malignancy, and liver failure, and is usually observed in hospitalised patients. It is characterised by systemic activation of blood coagulation leading to widespread fibrin deposition and the development of microvascular thrombi and may result in multiple organ dysfunction. The consumption of coagulation factors may subsequently induce severe bleeding.

Drugs

Patients with a history of cardiovascular disease are frequently prescribed anticoagulant drugs, such as warfarin, dabigatran, rivaroxaban, apixaban, and heparin. Anticoagulant therapy increases the risk of bleeding during oral surgical procedures. Nevertheless, minor surgical procedures, such as the extraction of up to three teeth, can be carried out safely using additional haemostatic measures in general dental practice settings. Patients on warfarin also need preoperative INR checks to ensure their INR is below 4.

Haemorrhage

Haemorrhage usually results from trauma or surgery and the response of the body is largely dependent on the severity of the blood loss (Table 16.3). Minor oral surgical procedures, such as tooth extractions, usually lead to minimal blood loss and are not accompanied by any significant cardiovascular changes. In contrast, severe and progressive blood loss may result from major trauma and surgery, which can lead to systemic hypoperfusion, owing to the reduction in cardiac output and/or reduction in effective circulatory blood volume (haemorrhagic shock).

Table 16.3 Classification of haemorrhage.

Parameter	Class 1	Class II	Class III	Class IV
Blood loss (ml)	750	750–1500	1500–2000	> 2000
Blood loss (%)	15	15–30	30–40	> 40
Heart rate (beats min^{-1})	< 100	100–120	120–140	> 140
Respiratory rate (breaths min^{-1})	< 20	20–30	30–40	> 35
Blood pressure	Normal	Normal	Decreased	Decreased
Urine output (ml h^{-1})	> 30	20–30	5–15	Negligible
CNS status	None	Anxiety	Confusion	Lethargy
Replacement requirements	None	Crystalloids/blood	Blood	Blood

To understand the body's response to blood loss (in the absence of medical intervention), it is customary to describe haemorrhagic shock in the following stages.

Stage I: Early Compensated Shock

If there is a minor deficiency in circulating blood volume, the following compensatory mechanisms are sufficient to maintain the cardiac output and blood pressure at near normal levels:

• Activation of sympathetic nervous system to increase the rate and force of heart contraction; constriction of peripheral arteriolar beds.
• Activation of the renin–angiotensin mechanism to increase aldosterone secretion.
• Increase in secretion of antidiuretic hormone.
• Increase in respiratory rate due to stimulation of peripheral chemoreceptors (increase in CO_2 and H^+ or a decrease in O_2). Baroreceptors in major vessels also increase respiratory rate in response to a drop in blood pressure (BP).

Stage II: Early Decompensated Shock

Persistence of shock, especially when accompanied by a further loss of blood, leads to a decline in cardiac output and BP. Tachypnoea as a result of decreased pulmonary perfusion is also common. Hypoxia may lead to a shift towards anaerobic glycolysis, production of lactic acid, and metabolic acidosis. However, the body tries to maintain perfusion to vital organs of the body at the expense of other organ systems.

Stage III: Progressive Decompensated Shock

Persistence of tissue hypoxia and worsening metabolic acidosis lead to microcirculatory changes with dilatation of arterioles while venules remain constricted. Pooling of blood in the tissues leads to stagnant hypoxia of the entire body: there is damage to the endothelium, leading to leakage of fluid and proteins into the tissues (oedema), impaired energy production, impaired membrane transport of ions, lysosomal enzyme leakage, and cell injury. Clinically, there is a progressive reduction in the cardiac output and BP. Ischaemia involving brain, heart, and kidneys leads to cell death in these organs with a progressively deepening coma.

Further Reading

Dr Najeeb Lectures (2018). Insulin: Synthesis and secretion: Part 1/4. https://www.youtube.com/watch?v=qGaTj8Scmrk (accessed 1 May 2018).

Hall, J.E. (2015). Chapter 37. In: *Guyton and Hall Textbook of Medical Physiology*, 13e. Philadelphia: Elsevier.

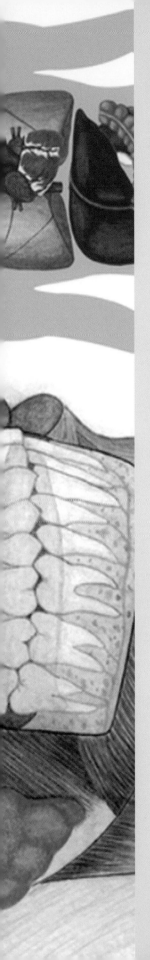

PART VIII
Endocrinology

CHAPTER 17
Endocrinology

Kamran Ali

Key Topics

- Overview of the pituitary, thyroid, and adrenal glands
- Common endocrine disorders ascsociated with these glands

Learning Objectives

To demonstrate an understanding of the:

- Chemical structure, functions, and control of hormones secreted by the pituitary, thyroid, and adrenal glands
- Causes and effects of hyper- and hyposecretion of pituitary, thyroid, and adrenal glands
- Relevance of common endocrine disorders to the provision of oral and dental care

Introduction

Hormones are secretions from glands and specialised cells *directly* into the blood. They produce a variety of effects on metabolism and growth. In this chapter we review the pituitary, thyroid, and adrenal glands.

Pituitary Gland (Hypophysis)

It is a pea-sized gland located in the hypophyseal fossa of the sphenoid bone in the middle cranial fossa. It is connected to the inferior aspect of the hypothalamus through the *hypophyseal stalk* (Figure 17.1). It is divided into two parts:

- Anterior pituitary (*adenohypophysis*): originates from an embryonic invagination of the pharyngeal epithelium and secretes several *peptide* hormones.

Essential Physiology for Dental Students, First Edition. Edited by Kamran Ali and Elizabeth Prabhakar.
© 2019 John Wiley & Sons Ltd. Published 2019 by John Wiley & Sons Ltd.
Companion website: www.wiley.com/go/ali/physiology

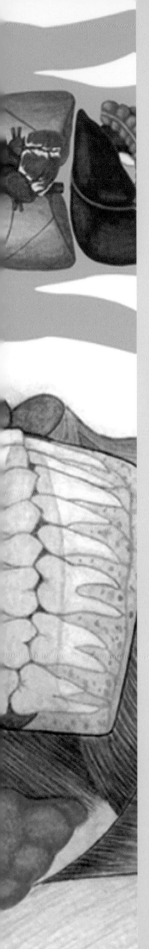

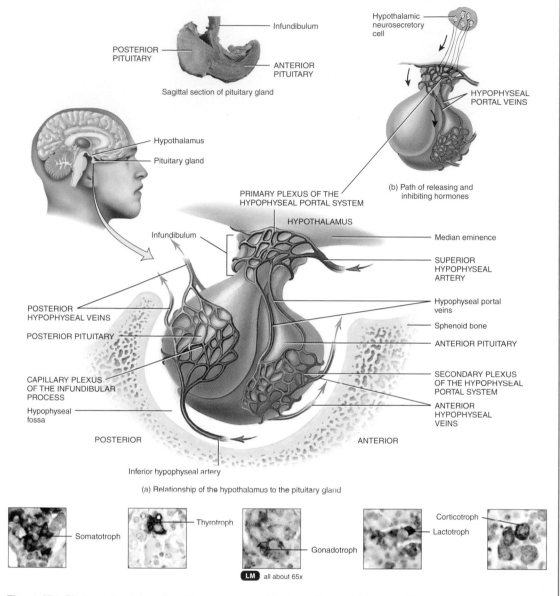

Figure 17.1 Pituitary gland: Location, blood supply and histology. *Source:* Tortora and Derrickson (2013).

• Posterior pituitary (*neurohypophysis*): originates from the lower end of the hypothalamus, is composed of neural tissue, and secretes two *peptide* hormones.

Anterior Pituitary Gland

The main hormones synthesised and secreted by the anterior pituitary are summarised along with their key actions in Table 17.1. These hormones are

Table 17.1 Hormones secreted by the anterior pituitary.

Hormone	Secretory Cells	Action	Regulation (Hypothalamus)	
			Stimulation	Inhibition
Growth hormone (GH)	Somatotrophs	Promotes generalised growth of the body	Growth-hormone-releasing hormone (GHRH)	Growth-hormone-inhibiting hormone (GHIH, somatostatin)
Adrenocorticotropic hormone (ACTH)	Corticotrophs	Stimulates adrenal cortex	Corticotropin-releasing hormone (CRH)	—
Thyroid stimulating hormone (TSH)	Thyrotrophs	Stimulates thyroid hormones (T3 and T4)	Thyrotropin-releasing hormone (TRH)	—
Prolactin hormone (PH)	Lactotrophs	Promotes mammary gland development and milk production	—	Prolactin-inhibiting hormone (PIH)
Gonadotropic hormones (GnH)	Gonadotrophs	Development of ovarian follicles Spermatogenesis in testis	Gonadotropin-releasing hormone (GnRH)	—
Follicle-stimulating hormone (FSH)		Ovulation		
Luteinising hormone (LH)		Production of sex hormones by ovaries and testis		

controlled by releasing and inhibitory factors secreted by the hypothalamus and transported to the anterior pituitary through the *hypothalamic–hypophyseal portal vessels*. All hormones from the anterior pituitary, except growth hormone (GH), exert their effects on specific target cells. In contrast, GH exerts its effects on the entire body.

Growth Hormone (Somatotropin)

GH is synthesised by specialised cells, called *somatotropes*, which constitute 30–40% of the cells in the anterior pituitary. The actions of GH include:

• Increases mitosis and size of cells throughout the body and promotes growth. These effects are particularly marked in skeletal tissues such as bone and cartilage. GH stimulates the liver to produce specific proteins, known as *somatomedins* (insulin-like growth factors), which enhance bone growth.

• Increased protein synthesis, which ultimately contributes to growth. GH specifically causes:
  ○ Increased transport of amino acids into the cells
  ○ Increased transcription of DNA in the nucleus
  ○ Increased RNA translation in ribosomes
  ○ Decreased breakdown of proteins.
• Increased breakdown and utilisation of fats.
• Decreased breakdown and utilisation of carbohydrates. This in turn increases blood glucose and stimulates insulin secretion. Excessive GH secretion can lead to *diabetogenic* effects predisposing the individual to type 2 diabetes (*pituitary diabetes*).

GH secretion is stimulated by growth-hormone-releasing hormone (GHRH) (hypothalamus), starvation (decreased blood glucose, free fatty acids, and proteins), exercise, and trauma. GH is inhibited by growth-hormone-inhibiting hormone

(GHIH) (hypothalamus), aging, obesity, and exogenous GH supplements.

Hypersecretion of GH in adolescence (before epiphyseal closure in long bones) leads to *gigantism*, which is characterised by increased height of the affected individual with an increased risk of secondary diabetes (as explained above).

Hypersecretion of GH in adults (after epiphyseal closure in long bones) leads to *acromegaly*, which is characterised by increased thickness of bones and soft tissues. Bone enlargement is particularly remarkable in the hands, feet, and craniofacial skeleton. Mandibular protrusion is characteristic and often requires surgical correction. Soft-tissue enlargement may manifest with macroglossia (enlarged tongue) and sialosis (enlarged salivary glands). Dental management may be complicated by diabetes and cardiac disease.

Hyposecretion of GH is usually associated with deficiency of other hormones of the anterior pituitary (panhypopituitarism). In children this leads to *dwarfism*, which is characterised by generalised growth retardation and lack of sexual development due to deficiency of GH and gonadotropins respectively. In adults, panhypopituitarism is characterised by deficiencies of thyroid, glucocorticoid and gonadotropin hormones. Dental management of patients with ACTH deficiency may be complicated by Addisonian crisis (described later).

Posterior Pituitary Gland

It secretes two peptide hormones, namely antidiuretic hormone (ADH) and oxytocin. These hormones are actually synthesised in the cell bodies of the *supraoptic* and *paraventricular* nuclei in the hypothalamus. ADH is primarily synthesised in the supraoptic, while oxytocin is formed in the paraventricular nucleus. The hormones are then transported in combination with carrier proteins (*neurophysins*) to the posterior pituitary through nerve tracks that traverse the pituitary stalk.

Antidiuretic Hormone (Vasopressin)

ADH conserves water by controlling the rate of water excretion in the urine. It increases the permeability of collecting ducts and tubules in the kidney to water. This leads to increased reabsorption of water in the renal tubules, resulting in excretion of a concentrated

urine. ADH (at high concentrations) also causes constriction of arterioles, with a resultant increase in arterial pressure, hence the name *vasopressin*.

ADH secretion is stimulated when the extracellular fluid (ECF) becomes concentrated to allow conservation of water (Figure 17.2). Conversely, when the ECF is diluted, the secretion of ADH is inhibited. Moreover, ADH secretion is stimulated by low blood volume and low blood pressure, for example following a haemorrhage.

Deficiency of ADH may lead to *diabetes insipidus*, which is characterised by excessive urination (polyuria), thirst, and dehydration. Xerostomia may be observed with it attendant complications.

Oxytocin

It causes powerful contraction of the uterus towards the end of gestation in pregnant subjects and induces labour. In addition, it facilitates lactation by promoting expression of milk from the alveoli into the ducts of the breast.

A synthetic analogue of oxytocin, known as *felypressin*, is used as a vasoconstrictor in dental local anaesthetics (in combination with prilocaine). Use of felypressin is best avoided in pregnant subjects, as there is a theoretical risk of premature induction of labour.

Thyroid Gland

The thyroid gland is located anterior to the trachea in the neck (Figure 17.3). It is shaped like a butterfly and consists of two lobes joined by a central isthmus. Weighing approximately 15–20 g, it is considered one of the largest endocrine gland. The thyroid gland develops as an epithelial proliferation at the base of the tongue between the *tuberculum impar* and the *copula*, a point demarcated later by the *foramen caecum*. The thyroid diverticulum then descends into the neck and divides into the lateral lobes and the isthmus.

The thyroid gland is composed of follicles lined by epithelium. The follicular cells secrete two hormones, namely triiodothyronine (T3) and tetra iodothyronine (T4, or thyroxine), which cause a marked increase in the metabolic rate. The parafollicular of *C cells* of the thyroid secrete another hormone, known as *calcitonin*, which has a role in calcium regulation and is discussed separately.

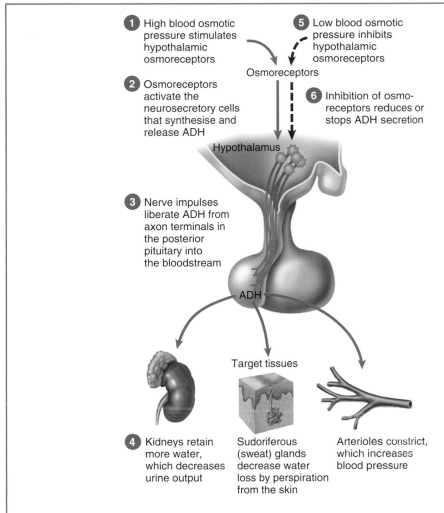

1. High blood osmotic pressure stimulates hypothalamic osmoreceptors

5. Low blood osmotic pressure inhibits hypothalamic osmoreceptors

Osmoreceptors

2. Osmoreceptors activate the neurosecretory cells that synthesise and release ADH

6. Inhibition of osmoreceptors reduces or stops ADH secretion

Hypothalamus

3. Nerve impulses liberate ADH from axon terminals in the posterior pituitary into the bloodstream

ADH

Target tissues

4. Kidneys retain more water, which decreases urine output

Sudoriferous (sweat) glands decrease water loss by perspiration from the skin

Arterioles constrict, which increases blood pressure

Figure 17.2 Control and actions of antidiuretic hormone secretion. *Source:* Tortora and Derrickson (2013).

Synthesis of Thyroid Hormones

The interior of the thyroid follicles is filled by a proteinaceous substance known as *colloid*. The main constituent of the colloid is *thyroglobulin*, a tyrosine-containing protein. The thyroid gland absorbs dietary iodine from the blood which is then oxidised to allow its coupling with tyrosine within the thyroglobulin molecules. Tyrosine is iodised successively to tri- and tetra-iodotyrosine, forming T3 and T4 hormones respectively. These remain stored as part of thyroglobulin within the colloid. Secretion of thyroid hormones involves their reabsorption from the follicles into the blood. Over 90% of thyroid hormones released into the blood consist of T4, but most of it is converted to T3 in the tissues.

Actions of Thyroid Hormones

Thyroid hormones produce marked effects on a number of cellular processes which result in an increased basal metabolic rate of the body.

At the cellular level, the actions of thyroid hormones lead to the following:

• Increased nuclear transcription of a large number of genes resulting in increased synthesis of proteins that function as enzymes, cell surface receptors, structural, and carrier proteins.

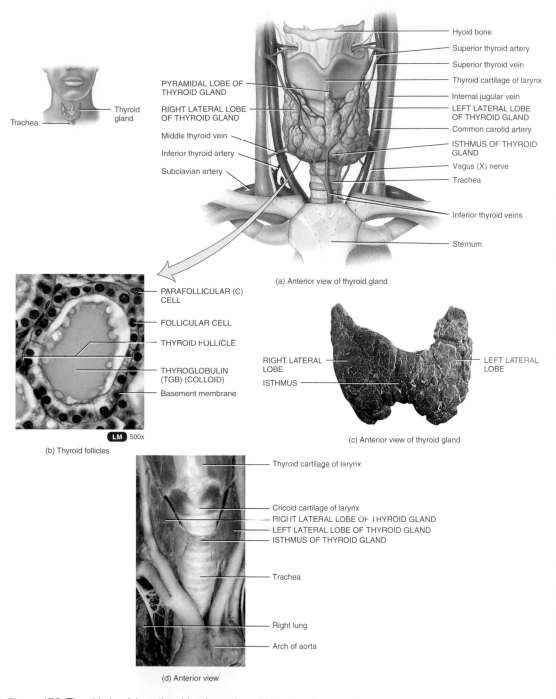

(a) Anterior view of thyroid gland

(b) Thyroid follicles

(c) Anterior view of thyroid gland

(d) Anterior view

Figure 17.3 Thyroid gland: Location, blood supply and histology. *Source:* Tortora and Derrickson (2013).

- Increased size and number of mitochondria.
- Increased rate of transport of ions across the cell membrane, including sodium and potassium.

The aforementioned effects lead to stimulation of a variety of metabolic activities:

- Increased carbohydrate metabolism, including glucose absorption from the gastrointestinal tract (GIT), cellular uptake of glucose, glycogenolysis, and gluconeogenesis.
- Increased fat metabolism, including their mobilisation from fat stores with a reduction in body weight. Plasma concentration and oxidation of free fatty acids is also increased. Secretion of cholesterol in the bile is also enhanced, which lowers its concentration in the plasma.
- Increased protein synthesis (in small amounts). Larger increases in thyroid hormones lead to protein catabolism, muscle weakness, and tremors.
- Increased utilisation of vitamins.

The increased metabolic activity resulting from thyroid hormones is complemented by a number of physiological effects:

- Increased rate and depth of respiration to compensate for increased demand of oxygen and the need to eliminate increased carbon dioxide resulting from metabolic activity. Dissociation of haemoglobin from oxyhaemoglobin is also enhanced, owing to increased production of 2,3-diphosphoglyceric acid.
- Increased heart rate, force of cardiac contraction, and cardiac output. The cardiovascular effects partly result from increased synthesis of adrenergic receptors by thyroid hormones which enhance the effect of sympathetic hormones.
- Increased motility of the GIT.

Finally, the thyroid hormones contribute to the growth of both skeletal as well as soft tissue, especially the brain. They are also required for normal sexual functions and menstruation.

Regulation of Thyroid Hormones

Synthesis and secretion of thyroid hormones is stimulated by TSH from the anterior pituitary, and TSH secretion itself is stimulated by TRH from the hypothalamus. As the hypothalamus regulates the central control of body temperature, exposure to cold stimulates TRH secretion. On the other hand, increased

levels of thyroid hormones suppress TSH secretion through a negative feedback. Thyroid secretion is also inhibited by antithyroid agents, such as thiocyanate, propyl thiouracil, and inorganic iodides.

Hyperthyroidism

The most-recognised form of hyperthyroidism is Grave's disease, which is an autoimmune disorder characterised by antibodies directed against the TSH receptors in the thyroid. These antibodies (thyroid stimulating immunoglobulins, or TSIs) simulate the actions of TSH and cause prolonged stimulation of the thyroid gland leading to its marked enlargement, or *goitre*. A typical feature of Grave's disease is exophthalmos (bulging of the eyeball), which is caused by oedema of retrobulbar tissues and degenerative changes in the extraocular muscles.

Adenomas (benign tumours) of the thyroid can cause excessive thyroid hormone production. The excessive levels of thyroid hormones inhibit TSH and may lead to atrophy of the remainder of the thyroid.

Hypothyroidism

Hypothyroidism may result from several causes and some of them are summarised below:

- *Endemic colloid goitre* results from dietary deficiency of iodine. Inadequate thyroid hormone synthesis leads to excessive TSH secretion, which stimulates the thyroid to produce large amounts of colloid (thyroglobulin), causing thyroid enlargement.
- *Non-toxic goitre* results from defects in enzymes required for iodine trapping and synthesis of thyroid hormones.
- *Hashimoto's thyroiditis* is an autoimmune disorder which causes destruction of the thyroid gland.
- *Cretinism* results from extreme congenital deficiency of thyroid hormones either due to genetic enzyme defects or dietary deficiency of iodine. It is characterised by impairment of physical (especially skeletal) growth and mental retardation. Macroglossia may develop with attendant difficulty in swallowing and breathing.
- *Myxoedema* is seen in adults with extreme thyroid deficiency and results to accumulation of hyaluronic acid and chondroitin sulphate in interstitial spaces, which impart a characteristic swelling of the face and bagginess under the eyes.

Table 17.2 Features of hyper- and hypothyroidism.

Hyperthyroidism	Hypothyroidism
Heat intolerance	Cold intolerance
Increased sweating	Reduced sweating
Warm moist skin	Cold, dry skin; hair loss
Irritability	Slow reactions
Insomnia	Somnolence
Muscles tremors	Hoarseness of voice
Increased appetite; diarrhoea	Reduced appetite; constipation
Weight loss	Weight gain
Tachycardia	Bradycardia
Atrial fibrillation; heart failure	Angina
Amenorrhoea; gynaecomastia	Menorrhagia

• *Iatrogenic* hypothyroidism follows surgical removal of thyroid as part of treatment for hyperthyroidism.

Owing to a close association of the development of the thyroid with the tongue, remnants of thyroid tissue may be found in the tongue (*lingual thyroid*) and it often presents as a lump between the foramen caecum and epiglottis.

The typical clinical features of hyper- and hyposecretion of thyroid hormones are summarised in Table 17.2.

Adrenal Gland

The adrenal glands are paired and located at the superior poles of the kidneys bilaterally (Figure 17.4). Each gland consists of an outer zone, known as the *adrenal cortex*, and an inner zone, known as the *adrenal medulla*. The adrenal cortex constitutes 80% of the gland and secretes several steroid hormones, all of which are synthesised from cholesterol. The adrenal medulla forms the remaining 20% of the gland and secretes two hormones (epinephrine and norepinephrine), which produce effects similar to those caused by stimulation of the sympathetic nerves and are discussed in Chapter 22.

Adrenal Cortex

The adrenal cortex consists of three distinct zones:

• *Zona glomerulosa* (outermost, thin zone): Secretes *mineralocorticoids*, which regulate sodium reabsorption and potassium excretion by the kidneys.

• *Zona fasciculata* (middle, widest zone): Secretes *glucocorticoids*, which regulate the body's response to stress and affect carbohydrate, protein, and lipid metabolism.
• *Zona reticularis* (innermost zone): Secretes *androgens*, which regulate sexual functions in males.

Glucocorticoids

The main glucocorticoid hormone secreted from the adrenal cortex in humans is *cortisol*. It helps the body to respond to stress and has several metabolic, anti-inflammatory, and antiallergic actions.

Actions

• *Carbohydrate metabolism:* Cortisol increases blood glucose levels by causing a multi-fold increase in gluconeogenesis and reducing glucose utilisation by cells. Excessive secretion cortisol can lead to *diabetogenic effects,* predisposing the individual to type 2 diabetes (*adrenal diabetes*).
• *Protein metabolism:* Cortisol increases protein breakdown in tissues and increases the mobilisation of amino acids in the blood, which are then utilised for protein synthesis in the liver, especially for the synthesis of plasma proteins.
• *Fat metabolism:* Cortisol increases mobilisation of fatty acids from adipose tissue by reducing the levels of α glycerophosphate. The increased free fatty acids in the plasma are then utilised for energy production. Obesity observed in hypersecretion of cortisol is perhaps related to increased appetite.

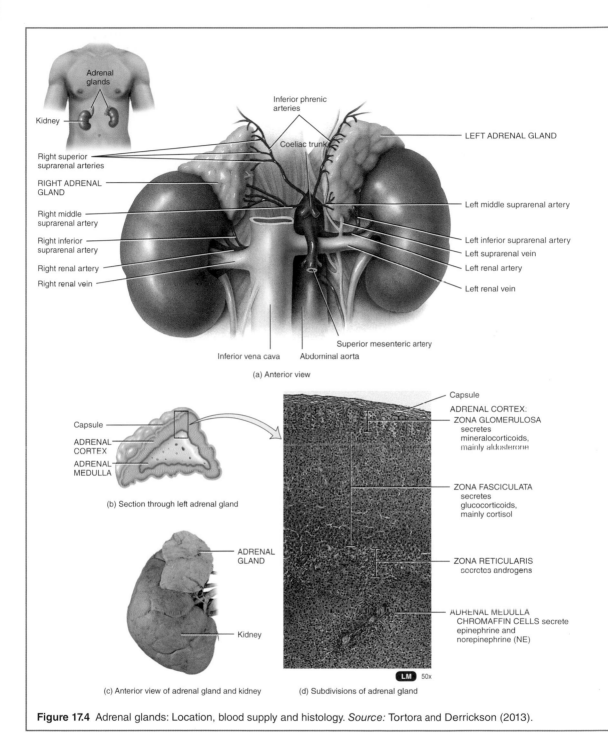

Figure 17.4 Adrenal glands: Location, blood supply and histology. *Source:* Tortora and Derrickson (2013).

• *Anti-inflammatory and immunosuppressive effects:* Cortisol has potent anti-inflammatory and antiallergic effects, owing to the following actions:

∘ Inhibition of phospholipase A2 to block the production of arachidonic acid metabolites, which are potent mediators of inflammation

○ Stabilisation of lysosomal membranes
○ Reduction in capillary permeability
○ Inhibitory effects on neutrophils, macrophages, and lymphocytes.

However, owing to its immunosuppressive effects, high levels of cortisol are associated with delayed wound healing and increased risk of opportunistic infections.

Regulation of Cortisol

Synthesis and secretion of cortisol is stimulated by ACTH from the anterior pituitary, which itself is stimulated by corticotropin-releasing hormone (CRH) from the hypothalamus. Stress caused by a variety of causes, such as trauma, surgery, and infection, stimulates secretion of ACTH. Increased cortisol levels (endogenous or exogenous) inhibit the secretion of ACTH and CRH through a negative feedback mechanism.

Disorders of Cortisol Secretion

Primary hypoadrenocorticism (Addison's disease) most commonly results from autoimmune damage but may also be caused by infection (tuberculosis), surgical removal, tumours, and drugs (rifampicin, ketoconazole). *Secondary hypoadrenocorticism* most commonly results from long-term steroid therapy.

The features of hypoadrenocorticism vary but usually include postural hypotension, fever, malaise, weakness, GIT symptoms (anorexia, nausea), weight loss, depression, impotence, and amenorrhoea.

Patients with primary hypoadrenocorticism may be at risk of Addisonian (steroid) crisis due to stress associated with dental interventions. The main issues include hypotension and hypoglycaemia due to reduced secretion of cortisol.

Hyperadrenocorticism may be caused by increased levels of ACTH from a pituitary tumour (Cushing's disease) or primary excess of cortisol from endogenous or exogenous source (Cushing's syndrome).

The features of hyperadrenocorticism include central fat deposition which may impart characteristic physical features, including a 'lemon on toothpick' appearance, moon face, and a buffalo hump (due to excess fat deposition at the back of the neck between the shoulders). Other features include hypertension, cardiac disease, secondary diabetes, atrophy of skin with easy bruising, frontal baldness in males, growth of facial hair (hirsutism), acne, osteoporosis, muscle weakness, reduced libido, psychosis, and depression.

Dental management of patients with hyperadrenocorticism may be complicated by hypertension, diabetes, psychosis, and cardiovascular disease. There is increased predisposition to opportunistic infections such as candidiasis due to immunosuppression. Surgical interventions like tooth extractions may be complicated by delayed wound healing and postoperative infection. Finally, patients on exogenous steroids may be at a theoretical risk of steroid crisis, owing to suppression of the adrenal–pituitary axis.

Mineralocorticoids

The main mineralocorticoid hormone secreted from the adrenal cortex in humans is aldosterone. The main function of aldosterone is to sustain the ECF volume by conserving sodium in the body and thereby maintaining venous return, cardiac output, and arterial blood pressure.

Actions

• The target tissue for aldosterone is the distal renal tubules, where it promotes active reabsorption of sodium by increasing the transcription of several transport proteins. Passive reabsorption of water follows sodium, allowing the isotonic expansion of ECF volume.
• It also stimulates active secretion of potassium into the lumen of the distal renal tubules and its ultimate excretion in the urine.

Regulation of Aldosterone

Synthesis and secretion of aldosterone is stimulated by:

• Activation of the renin–angiotensin system. Briefly, the juxtaglomerular cells of the kidney respond to hypovolemia by secreting *renin*, which acts on plasma *angiotensinogen* (secreted by liver) to form *angiotensin I*, which is further cleaved by angiotensin-converting enzyme (secreted by lungs) to *angiotensin II*. Angiotensin II stimulates the

secretion of aldosterone and also causes vasoconstriction. Both these actions help to raise arterial blood pressure.
- Increased plasma concentration of potassium.
- Reduced plasma concentration sodium.
- ACTH from the anterior pituitary (minor contribution).

Aldosterone synthesis is inhibited by atrial natriuretic peptide (ANP) secreted by atrial myocytes in response to volume expansion. ANP also inhibits activation of the renin–angiotensin system.

Disorders of Aldosterone Secretion

Primary hyperaldosteronism may be caused by an adrenal adenoma (Conn's syndrome) or bilateral adrenal hyperplasia. Secondary overproduction is seen in cardiac failure, renal artery stenosis, nephrotic syndrome, or liver cirrhosis. It is characterised by excessive retention of sodium with consequent hypertension and hypokalaemia.

Reference

Tortora, G.J. and Derrickson, B. (2013). *Principles of Anatomy and Physiology*. Hoboken, NJ: Wiley.

Further Reading

Hall, J.E. (2015). Chapters 76, 77, and 78. In: *Guyton and Hall Textbook of Medical Physiology*, 13e. Philadelphia: Elsevier.

Hasudungan, A. (2018). Endocrinology. https://www.youtube.com/watch?v=YcPicFL5Jnw (accessed 1 May 2018).

CHAPTER 18

Regulation of Blood Glucose

Kamran Ali

Key Topics

- Overview of blood glucose regulation
- Overview of diabetes mellitus

Learning Objectives

To demonstrate an understanding of the:

- Importance of blood glucose metabolism
- Role of insulin and glucagon in the maintenance of normal blood glucose levels
- Recognition of signs and symptoms of hypoglycaemia and hyperglycaemia
- Pathogenesis, complications, and diagnosis of diabetes mellitus
- Impact of diabetes mellitus on the provision of oral and dental care

Introduction

Glucose ($C_6H_{12}O_6$) is a monosaccharide and serves as a key source of energy for the human body. Glucose is oxidised through a series of chemical reactions to form adenosine triphosphate (ATP), which serves to meet the energy needs of the cells. Firstly, glucose breakdown in the cytoplasm, termed glycolysis, produces pyruvate. Later, pyruvate is oxidised within the mitochondria through the tricarboxylic acid cycle to yield ATP from adenosine diphosphate (ADP). Carbon dioxide and water are the products of glucose metabolism. The brain tissue relies exclusively on glucose for its energy needs (obligatory use) and uses approximately 1 mg of glucose per kg minute^{-1}, translating into 100–120 g per day in a 70 kg subject. Blood glucose concentration below 50 mg dl^{-1} may lead to hypoglycaemic shock.

Blood glucose concentration is regulated mainly by hormones secreted by the pancreas. The pancreas is a mixed gland with both exocrine and endocrine functions.

Essential Physiology for Dental Students, First Edition. Edited by Kamran Ali and Elizabeth Prabhakar.
© 2019 John Wiley & Sons Ltd. Published 2019 by John Wiley & Sons Ltd.
Companion website: www.wiley.com/go/ali/physiology

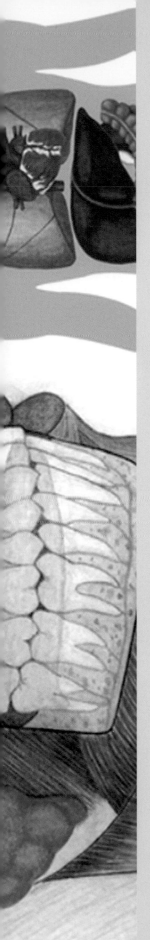

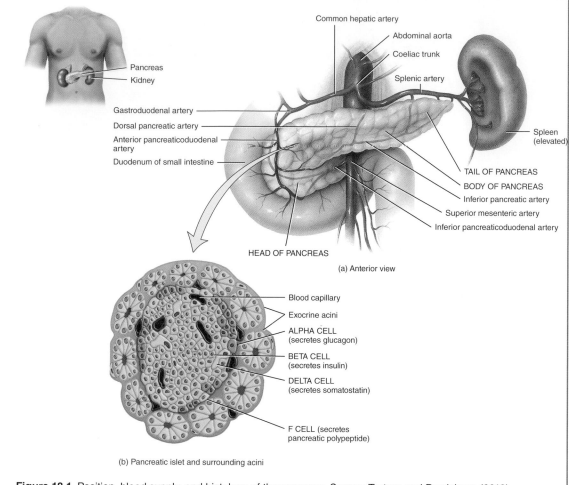

(a) Anterior view

(b) Pancreatic islet and surrounding acini

Figure 18.1 Position, blood supply, and histology of the pancreas. *Source:* Tortora and Derrickson (2013).

The exocrine pancreas consists of acinar cells which secrete pancreatic juice into the small intestine. The endocrine pancreas (islets of Langerhans) secretes insulin, glucagon, somatostatin, and pancreatic polypeptide (Figure 18.1). Blood glucose levels are reduced by insulin (primary hormone) and to a lesser extent by somatostatin. Blood glucose levels are increased by glucagon, adrenaline, noradrenaline, growth hormone, cortisol, and thyroxine.

Insulin

Insulin is a small protein secreted by ß cells which constitute 60% of endocrine pancreas. Insulin is composed of 51 amino acids arranged as a dimer with an A-chain and a B-chain linked together by disulfide bonds.

Functions of Insulin

Insulin exerts important effects on carbohydrate, protein, and fat metabolism, and these are summarised below:

- *Carbohydrate metabolism:* Insulin reduces blood glucose level in a number of ways:
  - Increased glucose uptake by almost all cells of the body, especially muscles, adipose tissue, and liver by increasing cell membrane permeability to glucose

○ Increased utilisation of glucose for energy production (especially during exercise), sparing fats, and proteins

○ Increased storage of glucose as glycogen in the liver by activation of the enzyme glycogen synthetase

○ Reduced gluconeogenesis in the liver

○ Increased uptake of glucose by the brain.

• *Protein metabolism:* Insulin is a protein-sparing hormone and reduces hepatic gluconeogenesis and also increases protein synthesis.

• *Fat metabolism:* Insulin reduces fat breakdown and promotes storage of fat into the adipose tissue by converting fatty acids into triglycerides.

Regulation of Insulin

Insulin secretion is stimulated mainly in response to high blood glucose levels. Other stimulants include the amino acids arginine and leucine; keto acids; acetylcholine; hormones, such as glucagon, adrenocorticotropic hormone (ACTH), growth hormone, and cortisol; and gastrointestinal tract (GIT) hormones, such as gastrin, secretin, and cholecystokinin. Insulin secretion is inhibited by stress-induced stimulation of adrenaline, hypoxia, and hypothermia.

Glucagon

Glucagon is a large polypeptide secreted by α cells, which constitute 25% of endocrine pancreas. It is a physiological antagonist of insulin and increases blood glucose levels.

Functions of Glucagon

Glucagon increases blood glucose concentration by stimulating the breakdown of liver glycogen (glycogenolysis) and increasing the rate of gluconeogenesis in the liver.

Due to its hyperglycaemic actions, glucagon is used to treat hypoglycaemia particularly if a patient has a reduced consciousness level and is unable to ingest sugary snacks or drinks.

Regulation of Glucagon

Glucagon secretion is stimulated mainly in response to low blood glucose levels. Other stimulants include the amino acids alanine and arginine, ß adrenergic stimulation (adrenaline and noradrenaline),

and cholecystokinin. Glucagon secretion is inhibited by insulin, somatostatin, increased fatty acids, ketones, and urea and alpha adrenergic (neural) stimulation.

Diabetes Mellitus

Diabetes mellitus (DM) is a group of metabolic disorders characterised by chronic hyperglycaemia. DM is one of the most common diseases worldwide and WHO figures show that the prevalence of diabetics has risen from 108 million in 1980 to 422 million in 2014. Any increase in blood glucose levels above the renal threshold (~10 mmol l^{-1} or 180 mg dl^{-1}) results in a failure of reabsorption of glucose from the renal tubules leading to *osmotic diuresis*, which causes loss of glucose and water in the urine. Therefore, diabetes frequently presents with polyuria (excessive urination), *polydipsia* (increase thirst due to dehydration), and *polyphagia* (increased hunger).

DM is traditionally classified into two main types:

• Type 1 diabetes has an autoimmune basis and leads to the destruction of ß cells in the pancreas, resulting in a lack of insulin production. Treatment of type 1 DM requires insulin, hence the old term *insulin-dependent diabetes.*

• Type 2 diabetes is characterised by relative deficiency of insulin resulting from either reduced production or resistance to insulin. Obesity and sedentary lifestyle are risk factors. Type 2 DM can be managed initially with diet control and lifestyle changes. However, long-term management often requires oral hypoglycaemics with or without insulin.

Impaired glucose tolerance (IGT) is an intermediate condition, often referred to as *pre-diabetes*, and poses a high risk of progressing to type 2 diabetes.

Gestational diabetes is seen during pregnancy due to high blood glucose levels.

Secondary causes of diabetes include endocrine disorders (hyperpituitarism, Cushing disease, pheochromocytoma), pancreatic disease (cystic fibrosis, haemochromatosis, chronic pancreatitis, pancreatectomy), liver cirrhosis, and drugs (e.g. corticosteroids), etc.

The diagnosis of diabetes in based on measurements of blood glucose levels, as shown in Table 18.1.

Long-term monitoring of blood glucose control may be done by measuring the levels of glycosylated haemoglobin (HbA1c), which

Table 18.1 Plasma glucose levels.

Plasma glucose test	Normal	Prediabetes	Diabetes
Random	Below 11.1 mmol l^{-1} Below 200 mg dl^{-1}	N/A	11.1 mmol l^{-1} or more 200 mg dl^{-1} or more
Fasting	Below 6.1 mmol l^{-1} Below 108 mg dl^{-1}	6.1–6.9 mmol l^{-1} 108–125 mg dl^{-1}	7.0 mmol l^{-1} or more 126 mg dl^{-1} or more
Two hours post-prandial	Below 7.8 mmol l^{-1} Below 140 mg dl^{-1}	7.8–11.0 mmol l^{-1} 140–199 mg dl	11.1 mmol l^{-1} or more 200 mg dl^{-1} or more

shows the blood glucose levels over the last 2-3 months based on the following criteria:

- Normal: Below 42 mmol mol^{-1} (6.0%)
- Prediabetes: 42–47 mmol mol^{-1} (6.0–6.4%)
- Diabetes: 48 mmol mol^{-1} (6.5% or more).

DM may present with a wide variety of symptoms and complications. Apart from polyuria, polydipsia, and polyphagia, DM may present acutely with diabetic ketoacidosis. Mainly seen in type 1 DM, ketoacidosis results from high blood glucose levels, leading to the production of ketone bodies and metabolic acidosis and presents with acetone breath, nausea, vomiting, dehydration, and hypotension. If untreated, it may progress to coma. Other presentations of DM may include weight loss, muscle cramps, weakness, fatigue, blurred vision, and skin infections.

Poorly controlled DM leads to major long-term complications with significant increase in morbidity and mortality. Blood vessels and nerves are the major target of DM. According to the WHO, DM is a major cause of blindness, kidney failure, heart attacks, stroke, lower limb amputation, and premature death.

Blood vessel damage may be related to advanced glycation end-products (AGEs) which result from glycation of fats and proteins through exposure to glucose. Blood vessel damage may involve several organ systems:

- *Retina:* DM leads to retinopathy with gradual vision loss and blindness.
- *Kidneys:* DM leads to nephropathy with protein loss and eventually chronic renal disease, often warranting renal dialysis and transplant.
- *Cardiovascular system:* DM increase atherosclerosis, increasing the risk of ischaemic heart disease, hypertension, and stroke.

Damage to the nerves (neuropathy) may lead to pain, altered or diminished sensation, muscle wasting, and dysfunction of the autonomic nervous system (postural hypotension, urinary incontinence, and impotence).

Neurovascular damage may also lead to chronic foot ulcers and gangrene, increasing the risk of foot/limb amputation.

Diabetes can be treated and its consequences avoided or delayed with dietary control, physical exercise, drugs, and regular screening and treatment for complications. Traditionally, management of DM is based on oral hypoglycaemic drugs, insulin, and homeopathic remedies. Modern treatments include pancreatic transplants and stem cell therapy.

Poorly controlled diabetics are at risk from several complications which may impact dental treatment and oral health:

- *Hypoglycaemia* is the most common medical emergency encountered in diabetics during dental appointments. The causes include missed, inadequate meals; overdose or inappropriate regimen of drugs, such as insulin; malabsorption; and alcohol intake. The dental professional must be able to recognise hypoglycaemia (Table 18.2), confirm blood glucose levels, and provide appropriate treatment to restore the blood glucose levels.

Chronic hyperglycaemia usually does not present as an emergency in dental practice but may lead to a number of oral manifestations:

- *Periodontal (gum) disease* is more common amongst diabetics and may result in premature tooth loss. There is emerging evidence that periodontal disease may also interfere with blood glucose control in diabetics, and its treatment may help improve blood glucose control.
- *Xerostomia* may result from dehydration with its attendant complications (see Section 10.2.3.1).
- *Delayed wound healing,* such as after a tooth extraction.

Table 18.2 Features of hypoglycaemia and hyperglycaemia.

Assessment	Hypoglycaemia	Hyperglycaemia
Causes1	Missed meals, insulin overdose, unusual exercise, malabsorption	Missed, insufficient insulin, excessive glucose intake
Onset	Rapid onset	Slow onset
Presentation	Irritability and aggression	Drowsiness and disorientation
	Moist sweaty skin	Dry skin, dry mouth
	Pulse full and rapid	Pulse weak and rapid
	Dysarthria	Acetone breath; ketonuria
	Normal or high blood pressure	Hypotension
	Headache; neurological fits	Abdominal pain
	Normal or shallow breathing	Hyperventilation
	Loss of consciousness (rapid)	Loss of consciousness (slow)
Glucose measurements	Blood sugar low [Usually < 3.0 mmol/l^{-1} (54 mg dl^{-1})]	Blood sugar high [Usually > 20 mmol l^{-1} (360 mg dl^{-1})]
	Urine sugar absent	Urine sugar usually present

• *Opportunistic infections.* One of the most common oral infection is caused by the fungus *Candida*. Several forms of oral *candidiasis* may be seen. Denture sore mouth (chronic atrophic candidiasis) is seen in patients wearing full upper dentures and is characterised by erythema of the palate, mirroring the denture base. Angular cheilitis causes cracking and bleeding around the corners of the mouth and may be causes by candidal and/or staphylococcal infection in patients wearing full dentures with reduced vertical dimensions.

Lastly, dental care in diabetics may be complicated by other coexisting complications, such as cardiovascular, renal, and neurological disease(s) requiring additional precautions in consultation with the patient's physicians.

Reference
Tortora, G.J. and Derrickson, B.H. (2013). *Principles of Anatomy and Physiology*, 14e. Hoboken, NJ: Wiley.

Further Reading
Diabetes.co.uk (2018). The global diabetes community. http://www.diabetes.co.uk.
Dr Najeeb Lectures (2018). Insulin: Synthesis and secretion: Part 1/4. https://www.youtube.com/watch?v=qGaTj8Semrk (accessed 1 May 2018).
Hall, J.E. (2015). Chapter 79. In: *Guyton and Hall Textbook of Medical Physiology*, 13e. Philadelphia: Elsevier.

CHAPTER 19

Regulation of Blood Calcium

Kamran Ali

Key Topics

- Overview of the role of calcium in the human body
- Regulation of blood calcium level

Learning Objectives

To demonstrate an understanding of the:

- Distribution of calcium in mineralised tissues and body fluids
- Role of vitamin D, parathormone, and calcitonin in calcium homeostasis
- Common disorders of calcium metabolism and their relevance to the provision of oral care

Introduction

Calcium is an essential mineral which provides structural integrity to mineralised tissues of the body (bones and teeth) and also plays a key role in a number of important physiological processes in the body. Calcium ions in extracellular and cellular fluids are essential to a host of biochemical processes, including neuromuscular excitability, hormonal secretion (second messenger), enzymatic regulation, blood coagulation, and exocytosis.

Most of the calcium in the body (99%) is stored in the bones and teeth in the form of hydroxyapatite. The bone mass of the body is mainly composed of cortical bone (80%), and only 20% is trabecular bone. However, trabecular bone has five times the surface area and is more important to calcium turnover.

Essential Physiology for Dental Students, First Edition. Edited by Kamran Ali and Elizabeth Prabhakar.
© 2019 John Wiley & Sons Ltd. Published 2019 by John Wiley & Sons Ltd.
Companion website: www.wiley.com/go/ali/physiology

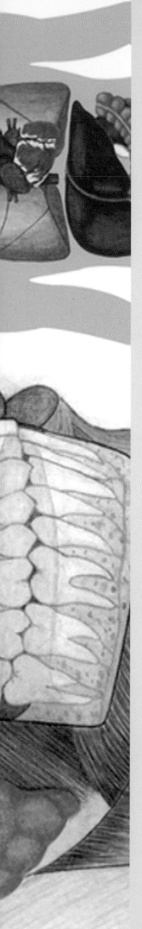

Plasma calcium concentration is regulated narrowly and normally ranges from 2.2 to 2.6 mmol l^{-1} (average 2.4 mmol l^{-1}). There are three definable fractions of calcium in the plasma:

- *Ionised calcium* 50% 1.2 mmol l^{-1}
  - This is the *physiologically relevant* fraction of calcium and contributes to most actions of calcium.
- *Protein-bound calcium* 40% (1.0 mmol l^{-1})
  - This fraction is primarily bound to albumin (90%); the remainder is bound to globulins. The binding of calcium to albumin is pH dependent. Acute alkalosis increases calcium binding to protein and decreases ionised calcium.
- *Complexed to serum constituents* 10% (0.2 mmol l^{-1})
  - This fraction is complexed with citrate and phosphate.

Intracellular calcium is stored in the mitochondria and the endoplasmic reticulum and is approximately 1/1000th of its concentration in the extracellular fluids.

Three principal hormones regulate calcium and three organs play an important function in calcium homeostasis. Parathyroid hormone (PTH), vitamin D, and calcitonin regulate calcium resorption, absorption, and excretion from the bone, intestine, and the kidneys respectively. In addition, many other hormones affect bone formation and resorption.

Disorders of Calcium

Hypercalcaemia

Raised levels of plasma calcium (> 2.6 mmol l^{-1}) may be associated with alkalosis, hyperparathyroidism, bone cancer, vitamin D toxicity, Paget's disease, hypothyroidism, and medications (e.g. lithium and hydrochlorothiazide).

Hypercalcaemia leads to reduced membrane permeability to sodium and inhibits depolarisation. Concentrations above 12 mEq l^{-1} cause muscular weakness, depressed reflexes, and cardiac arrhythmias. Cardiac arrest and coma may be seen in severe cases. Other symptoms may be related to the primary cause of hypercalcaemia (see Sections 19.4.4 and 19.5.2.1.1).

Hypocalcaemia

Common causes of low plasma calcium (< 2.1 mmol l^{-1}) include vitamin D deficiency, hypoparathyroidism, diarrhoea, pregnancy, lactation, kidney failure,

hyperthyroidism, and medications (e.g. overdose of calcium channel blockers and bisphosphonates).

Hypocalcaemia results in increased membrane permeability to sodium, which leads to nerve hyperexcitability, causing neuromuscular hyperexcitability; very low levels result in tetany, laryngospasm, and death. Two classic signs associated with hypocalcaemia include:

- *Trousseau's sign:* Inflating the blood pressure cuff to a level above systolic pressure for three minutes results in carpopedal spasm (a painful cramp in the muscles of hands and feet). This can be observed before the development of hyperreflexia and tetany as a result of hypocalcaemia.
- *Chvostek's sign:* Tapping the area innervated by the facial nerve leads to twitching of facial muscles.

Sometimes, anxiety associated with dental appointments may result in a *hyperventilation syndrome* characterised by quick, shallow breaths from the top of the chest. These quick, shallow breaths reduce the level of carbon dioxide (P_{CO_2}) in the blood. This reduced level of carbon dioxide causes the arteries to constrict, reducing the flow of blood throughout the body. When this occurs, our brain and body will experience a shortage of oxygen. Moreover, reduced levels of carbon dioxide in the blood may lead to respiratory alkalosis, resulting in increased binding of calcium to plasma proteins with resultant hypocalcaemia. The affected subject may experience tingling in the fingers and toes along with painful muscle spasm. Rebreathing with the hands covering the nostrils raises blood carbon dioxide levels and may help reverse the symptoms.

Vitamin D

Humans may acquire vitamin D (cholecalciferol) from dietary sources as well as *de novo* synthesis from the activation of the vitamin D precursor in the skin by absorption of ultraviolet radiation. The keratinocytes store 7-dehydrocholesterol which is activated by ultraviolet radiation to form cholecalciferol (Figure 19.1).

Vitamin D itself is inactive and requires modification to 1,25-dihydroxy cholecalciferol [1,25-(OH)$_2$-D]. The first hydroxylation occurs in the liver, yielding 25 HCC. The second hydroxylation occurs in the kidney (stimulated by parathormone) forming 1,25-(OH)$_2$-D. Vitamin D, after its activation to the hormone 1,25-(OH)$_2$-D, is a principal regulator of

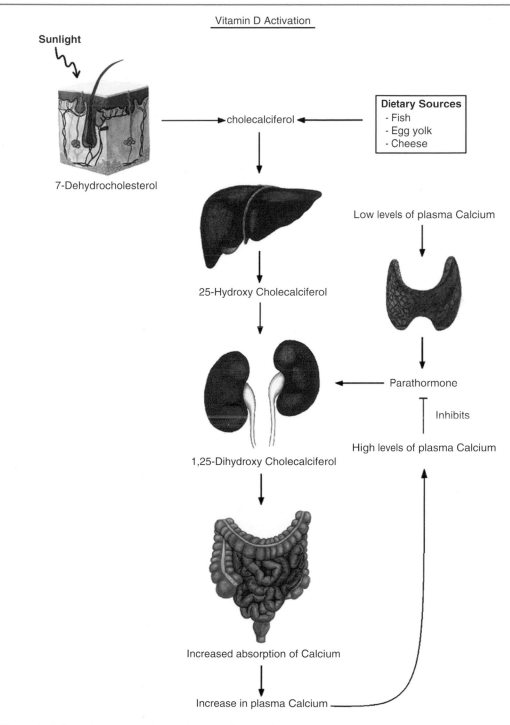

Vitamin D Activation

Figure 19.1 Steps in the activation of vitamin D. *Source:* Courtesy of Melina S.Y. Kam.

calcium. Evidence also suggests that keratinocytes in the skin are not only capable of synthesising cholecalciferol as described above but can also lead to its activation into $1,25\text{-}(OH)_2\text{-}D$ independently from the kidneys.

$1,25\text{-}(OH)_2\text{-}D$ is not considered a classic hormone, as it is not secreted by an endocrine gland. Nevertheless, its action is similar to that of hormones as it acts on distant target cells to evoke responses after binding to high-affinity receptors. It regulates plasma calcium by the principal mechanisms:

• It increases calcium absorption from intestinal epithelium by stimulating several calcium-binding proteins (as shown in Figure 19.1).
• It regulates bone formation. Osteoblasts, but not osteoclasts, have vitamin D receptors. $1,25\text{-}(OH)_2\text{-}D$ acts on osteoblasts, which produce a paracrine signal that activates osteoclasts to resorb Ca^{2+} from the bone matrix. It also stimulates osteocytic osteolysis.

Disorders of Vitamin D

Hypovitaminosis D

Prolonged deficiency of dietary vitamin D, intestinal malabsorption, and/or reduced exposure to sunlight may lead to excess osteoid accumulation from repression of osteoblastic collagen synthesis. The softening of bones (and associated deformities) due to vitamin D deficiency is referred to as *rickets* in children and *osteomalacia* in adults. Although vitamin D is widely available, a deficiency of vitamin D remains a problem for children and adults in underdeveloped countries as well as amongst the elderly in developed countries.

Rickets

Rickets affects children and is characterised by inadequately mineralised bones, causing softening and weakening of bones. Bowed legs and deformities of the pelvis, skull, and rib cage are common. Some characteristic features of rickets include:

• *craniotabes* (thin, deformed skull)
• *rickety rosary* (beading at costochondral junctions)
• *Harrison's sulcus* (groove at the lower end of the rib cage).

Dentition may also show signs of hypomineralisation.

Osteomalacia

Osteomalacia affects adults and often leads to softened, inadequately mineralised bones. Deformities of the spine, bowing of the legs, musculoskeletal pain, and increased risk of fractures are common.

Hypervitaminosis D

Excess of vitamin D is rare and usually related to a high intake of vitamin D supplements. It is characterised by features of hypercalcaemia with gastrointestinal tract symptoms (anorexia, nausea, vomiting, and diarrhoea), polyuria, polydipsia, insomnia, and nervousness. Long-term complications include metastatic calcifications and risk of renal failure.

Parathormone

Parathyroid hormone (PTH) is produced by small parathyroid glands located in the neck on the posterior aspect of the thyroid gland. Humans usually have four parathyroid glands with two glands located bilaterally on the superior and inferior thyroid lobes. The two superior glands arise from the epithelial lining of the fourth pharyngeal pouch, and the two inferior glands arise from the third pouch before occupying their final position. The parathyroid glands share their blood supply and lymphatic drainage with the thyroid gland (Figure 19.2).

Actions of the PTH

The PTH increases plasma calcium and decreases plasma phosphate levels by several mechanisms, including:

• Acts directly on the bones to stimulate Ca^{2+} resorption.
• Acts directly on the kidney to stimulate Ca^{2+} reabsorption in distal renal tubules and to inhibit reabsorption of phosphate (stimulating its excretion).
• Stimulates $1,25\text{-}(OH)_2\text{-}D$ synthesis and indirectly enhances the absorption of calcium from the intestine.

Regulation of PTH

Plasma calcium regulates PTH secretion through a negative feedback. Maximum secretion of PTH occurs at plasma Ca^{2+} below $3.5\,mg\,dl^{-1}$ within

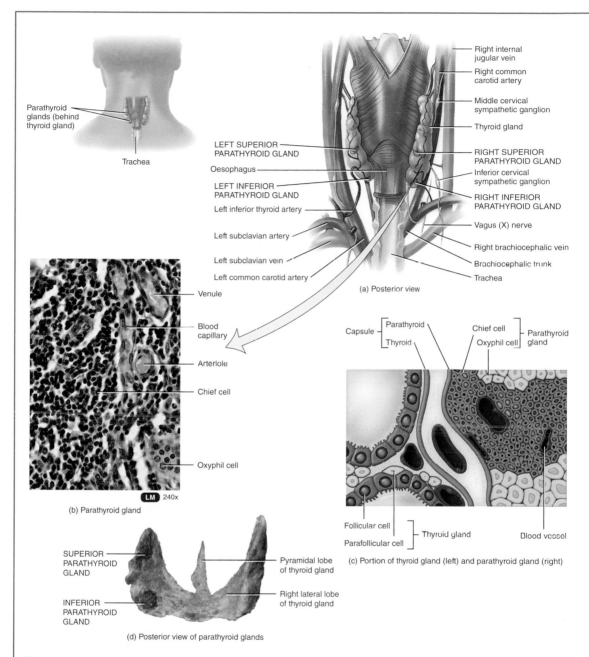

Figure 19.2 Location, blood supply, and histology of parathyroid glands. *Source:* Tortora and Derrickson (2013).

seconds (via cyclic adenosine monophosphate, or cAMP). At Ca^{2+} above $5.5\,mg\,dl^{-1}$, PTH secretion is maximally inhibited. Plasma phosphate levels have no direct effect on PTH secretion. $1,25\text{-}(OH)_2\text{-}D$ inhibits PTH gene expression, providing another level of feedback control of PTH.

Disorders of Parathyroid Gland

Hyperparathyroidism

• *Primary:* Caused by parathyroid tumours; leads to increased levels of serum PTH and calcium.

- *Secondary:* Results from chronic renal failure and malabsorption of vitamin D. It is characterised by reduced serum calcium and raised PTH levels.
- *Tertiary:* Results from adenoma formation in the parathyroids due to continuous stimulation of PTH secretion in secondary form.

Hyperparathyroidism is asymptomatic in 50% of cases. Generalised decalcification of the bones may result from calcium resorption and sometimes leads to lytic lesions in the bone, simulating a cyst. Hypercalcaemia also increases the risk of nephrocalcinosis and renal stones, which may in turn affect the renal function. Calcification of soft tissues, cornea, and blood vessels may also be seen. Other manifestations include dyspepsia, pruritus, myopathy, cardiac arrhythmias, and psychiatric disorders.

Hyperparathyroidism may lead to jaw bone resorption, resulting in generalised bone rarefaction and loss of lamina dura. Lytic bone lesions (usually multiple) may be identified on routine radiographs. Microscopically, these lesions display multinucleated giant cells and are often misinterpreted as jaw cysts.

Hypoparathyroidism

- *Postoperative:* Develops as a complication of thyroidectomy in up to 1% of cases.
- *Infantile:* May be caused by maternal deficiency of PTH or calcium and is usually transient. However, when associated with thymic aplasia (DiGeorge syndrome), it is permanent.
- *Idiopathic:* No known cause but may possibly result from autoimmune damage and can develop at any age.
- *Pseudohypoparathyroidism:* Congenital variety due to tissue resistance to PTH (defective post-receptor mechanism). Characterised by elevated PTH; mental retardation; resistance to TSH, glucagon and gonadotropins; and skeletal abnormalities, such as small stature; and short fourth and fifth metatarsals and metacarpals.
- *Pseudo-pseudohypoparathyroidism:* Skeletal abnormalities as with pseudo type but normal serum calcium.

Hypoparathyroidism may present with signs of hypocalcaemia, which have been discussed earlier. In addition, have several manifestations including epilepsy, myopathy, arrhythmias, tetany, mental handicap, and psychiatric problems. It may also be associated with hypoadrenocorticism and diabetes mellitus (DM).

Oral manifestations may include enamel hypoplasia, shortened dental roots, chronic mucocutaneous candidiasis (fungal infection), and facial paraesthesia.

Calcitonin

Calcitonin is synthesised and secreted by parafollicular cells of the thyroid gland which can be distinguished from follicular cells of the thyroid gland by their large size, pale cytoplasm, and smaller secretory granules.

Actions of Calcitonin

Calcitonin acts to decrease plasma calcium levels and is a physiological antagonist to PTH with regard to calcium homeostasis.

Regulation of Calcitonin

The major stimulus of calcitonin secretion is a rise in plasma Ca^{2+} levels. It targets the osteoclasts and acts to inactivate osteoclasts, which results in the rapid inhibition of bone resorption. However, PTH and vitamin D3 regulation dominate in the overall control serum calcium. Chronic hypersecretion of calcitonin is not associated with hypocalcaemia, and nor does the removal of parafollicular cells cause hypercalcaemia. Perhaps calcitonin plays a more important role in regulating bone remodelling than in calcium homeostasis.

Reference

Tortora, G.J. and Derrickson, B. (2013). *Principles of Anatomy and Physiology*. Hoboken, NJ: Wiley.

Further Reading

Hall, J.E. (2015). Chapter 80. In: *Guyton and Hall Textbook of Medical Physiology*, 13e. Philadelphia: Elsevier.
Hasudungan, A. (2018). Endocrinology: Calcium and phosphate regulation. https://www.youtube.com/watch?v=EEM0iRJNhU8 (accessed 1 May 2018).

CHAPTER 20

Reproductive Hormones and Pregnancy

Theresa Compton and Kamran Ali

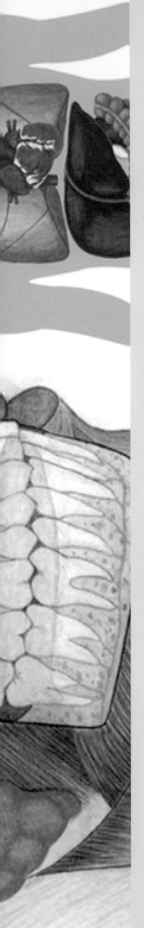

Key Topics

- Organisation of the male and female reproductive systems
- Overview of the female reproductive cycle and pregnancy

Learning Objectives

To demonstrate an understanding of the:

- Structure of male and female reproductive organs
- Role of hormones in ovarian cycle and pregnancy
- Physiological changes in pregnancy
- Impact of pregnancy on the provision of dental care

Organisation of the Reproductive Tract

The female reproductive tract consists of the uterus, cervix, fallopian (uterine) tubes, ovaries, vagina, and external genitalia (Figure 20.1). Arising from fusion of the paramesonephic ducts, the uterus is a muscular pear-shaped organ that contains and protects the developing foetus, while the cervix (the neck of the uterus) has an important role in reproduction of protecting the developing foetus from infection and premature delivery. Developing from the peritoneum, the ovaries are made up of the ova (developing gametes) and the supporting theca and granulosa cells. These produce hormones under the influence of the hypothalamic–pituitary axis. The fallopian tubes collect the mature ovum and transport it to the uterus.

The male reproductive tract comprises the penis and testes. The testes are the site of development of the sperm, and have equivalent supporting cells to the theca and granulosa cells in the female – the leydig and sertoli cells. Erection of the penis is required for delivery of sperm adjacent to the cervix. Approximately 99% of sperm

Essential Physiology for Dental Students, First Edition. Edited by Kamran Ali and Elizabeth Prabhakar.
© 2019 John Wiley & Sons Ltd. Published 2019 by John Wiley & Sons Ltd.
Companion website: www.wiley.com/go/ali/physiology

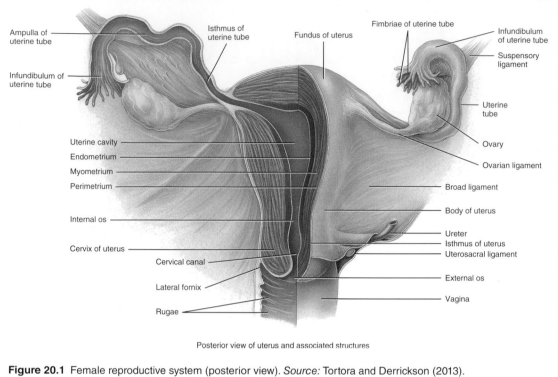

Ampulla of uterine tube

Infundibulum of uterine tube

Isthmus of uterine tube

Fundus of uterus

Fimbriae of uterine tube

Infundibulum of uterine tube

Suspensory ligament

Uterine tube

Ovary

Ovarian ligament

Broad ligament

Body of uterus

Ureter
Isthmus of uterus
Uterosacral ligament

External os

Vagina

Uterine cavity
Endometrium
Myometrium
Perimetrium

Internal os

Cervix of uterus

Cervical canal

Lateral fornix

Rugae

Posterior view of uterus and associated structures

Figure 20.1 Female reproductive system (posterior view). *Source:* Tortora and Derrickson (2013).

are caught in the cervix or cervical mucous, with 1% making it into the uterus. Sperm can survive for approximately seven days in the female reproductive tract.

Monthly Ovarian Cycle

During the reproductive years, the female reproductive system is prepared for conception and pregnancy. Each monthly cycle in the female lasts for approximately 28 days and involves physical changes in the female reproductive tract under the influence of hormones. The gonadotropic hormones from the anterior pituitary lead to the development of new follicles in the ovaries (follicular phase). The secretory cells of the ovum (egg) develop into corpus luteum, which secretes the female hormones. If the ovum meets a sperm, it may become fertilised and initiate pregnancy. If the ovum is not fertilised, the female hormone levels decrease, leading to degeneration of the corpus luteum over the remaining 14 days (luteal phase), followed by menstruation.

Hormonal Secretions by the Hypothalamic–Pituitary Axis

Events in the ovary and endometrium are under the central control of hormones from the hypothalamus and pituitary in the brain, as shown in Figure 20.2. Gonadotrophin-releasing hormone produced from the hypothalamus initiates the release of *luteinising hormone* (LH) and *follicle-stimulating hormone* (FSH) from the pituitary. These stimulate cells in the ovary to produce *oestrogen* (oestradiol) and *progesterone*, which exert their effects on the endometrium (and other targets). *Activin* produced in the ovary potentiates the effect of FSH, whereas *inhibin*, another hormone, downregulates FSH action and exerts negative feedback on the pituitary.

Ovulation

Normally, a single ovum is released from one of the ovaries each month. Multiple follicles develop in the ovary, each one consisting of the ovum, surrounding granulosa cells, and theca cells.

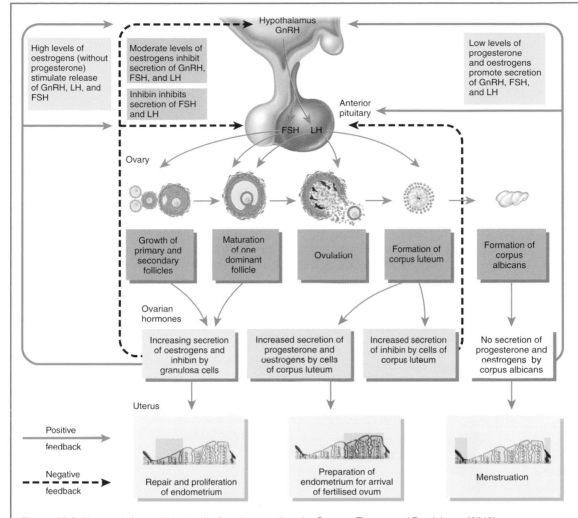

Figure 20.2 Hormonal interactions in the female sexual cycle. *Source:* Tortora and Derrickson (2013).

A successful follicle, containing a fluid-filled antrum, is selected for ovulation and protrudes from the surface of the ovary. The remaining follicles degenerate. LH stimulates theca cells to produce androgens from cholesterol via steroidogenesis. Granulosa cells proliferate in response to FSH, and these convert the androgens from the theca cells into oestrogen. As the ovum ruptures out of the ovary, it is collected by the fimbriae of the fallopian tube. After ovulation, the egg survives for just one day. The remaining granulosa cells form the corpus luteum – a part of the ovary that continues to produce oestrogen and progesterone. If fertilisation occurs, the corpus luteum will persist under the

action of human chorionic gonadotrophin (hCG), a hormone produced by the developing trophoblast. If fertilisation does not occur the corpus luteum will degenerate, and the cycle will begin again. A protein in sperm, catsper, can detect progesterone produced by the corpus luteum, which in turn, increases motility of the sperms tail, allowing it to move towards the released ovum.

Transport of Ovum

Eggs are collected by the fimbriae of the fallopian tubes via chemotaxis. Ciliated cells facilitate interactions between the egg and the fallopian tube and allow the propulsion of the egg towards the uterus. Peg cells in the fallopian tube produce fluid that supports the growing embryo and enables sperm survival, with the majority of fertilisations taking place here.

Fertilisation

In meeting a sperm, the egg may become fertilised. The head of the sperm, or acrosome, contains acrosin and hyaluronidase enzymes to facilitate passage through the corona radiata of the egg (outer granulosa cells) and permeation of the zona pellucida, the thick outer layer of the ovum, to allow fusion of the two gametes.

Once completed, cell division begins in two-cell, four-cell stages, until a morula (berry appearance) stage is reached. Disintegration of the zona pellucida permits the entry of fluid into the centre of the bundle of cells, creating a blastocyst. The cells then specialise to form an embryoblast, which becomes the developing embryo, and the trophoblast, which invades the endometrium to become the developing placenta.

Uterus and Endometrium

The uterus is the site for development of an embryo and consists of three layers: the inner *endometrium*, which is shed during menstruation; the *myometrium* or muscle layer, which contracts in labour and at menses; and the outer *perimetrium*, which provides a peritoneal covering. In the menstrual cycle the lining of the endometrium thickens and sheds in relation to the concentration of the oestrogen and progesterone.

Oestrogen appears to exert a proliferative effect on endometrial tissues, with five days of oestrogenic exposure producing tissue thick enough for implantation. Progesterone halts proliferation and changes the functionality of endometrial stromal cells to accumulate glycogen and produce cytokines and extracellular matrix proteins, a process called *decidualisation*. Decidualisation seems to be important in protecting the mother from trophoblast invasion, and in the development of a healthy pregnancy.

Pregnancy

As the trophoblast embeds into the endometrium, it produces a number of hormones that support and establish the developing pregnancy, taking over from the corpus luteum (Table 20.1). Initially, hCG enables invasion of the trophoblast and is the one that pregnancy tests detect. It has been implicated in morning sickness and the polyuria that women experience. Oestrogen produced by the fetoplacental unit results in angiogenesis of uterine vessels, and myometrial growth. Progesterone has been implicated in immune tolerance and prevents rejection of the foetus by the maternal immune system.

Labour and Contractions

During labour, oestrogen and progesterone's actions on the oxytocin receptor are antagonistic – with oestrogen promoting contractions, and progesterone preventing them, and prolonging gestation. Oestrogen

Table 20.1 Role of placental hormones in pregnancy.

Hormones produced by placenta	Role
hCG	Prolongs the corpus luteum, which in turn produces oestrogen and progesterone to support the pregnancy
Progesterone	Prevention of contraction, smooth muscle relaxation, immunity
Oestrogen	Growth of tissues, gap junctions, promotes contractions during labour
Relaxins	Softening of cervix
Human placental lactogen/ somatomammotropin	Acts as an anti-insulin, and increases the amount of circulating glucose available for the foetus.
Corticotrophin-releasing hormone	Enables foetus to produce cortisol, which stimulates type 2 pneumocytes to produce surfactant, readying the foetal lungs for the first breath
Oxytocin	Contractions in labour, let down reflex

promotes an increase in the number of gap junctions between myometrial cells, allowing waves of contraction to spread easily. Progesterone acts as a smooth muscle relaxant, not only on the uterus but also on other smooth muscle, which has consequences in the urinary tract, gastrointestinal tract, and vessels.

Physiologic Changes During Pregnancy

Systemic physiological changes in pregnancy give an understanding of the potential clinical problems with pregnancy, including likely risk factors for mortality, such as sepsis and venous thromboembolism.

Respiratory Changes During Pregnancy

Pregnancy increases the oxygen requirements by approximately 15%. Hypoxaemia may lead to breathlessness, particularly in the supine position. This is compensated by hyperventilation and upward displacement of the diaphragm by 2–4 cm. Nevertheless, breathlessness during pregnancy must be investigated to rule out a cardiac cause. Pregnant women may find dental treatment in a supine position particularly difficult in the third trimester.

Cardiovascular Changes During Pregnancy

During pregnancy, there is a 20–30% increase in heart rate as well as a 20–50% increase in stroke volume. As a result, the cardiac output increases by 30–50% secondary to volume. Moreover, the peripheral vascular resistance is decreased during pregnancy, owing to peripheral vasodilatation. Therefore, pregnant women receiving dental treatment in a supine position are susceptible to postural hypotension when standing up, which may lead to fainting.

Pregnancy leads to an enormous growth of the uterus, which may increase from 50 g pre-pregnancy to 1000 g at term. This progressively decreases the space for other abdominal organs. During the third trimester, the uterus may compress the inferior vena cava and aorta when the subject is supine. This may lead to a reduction in cardiac output as well as blood pressure. Placing the subject in a 5–15° tilt on the left side in the dental chair may relieve venous compression and improve circulation during dental treatment. If symptoms are not relieved, a full left lateral position may be required.

Gastrointestinal Tract

Enlargement of the uterus causes displacement of the stomach towards the spleen and liver, raising the intragastric pressure. Progesterone inhibits the hormone motilin, which decreases the lower oesophageal sphincter tone and also slows gastric emptying. These changes lead to pyrosis (heartburn), regurgitation, gastro-oesophageal reflux disease, and hyperemesis. Surgery on pregnant women under general anaesthesia is associated with increased risk of aspiration, which can be fatal.

Gastro-oesophageal reflux disease during pregnancy can lead to marked tooth surface loss due to dental erosion. Furthermore, women may also experience increased sugar cravings, increasing the risk of tooth decay.

Oral tissues are sensitive to hormones and rich in receptors for oestrogen and progesterone, which can lead to localised overgrowth of gingival tissues, termed *pyogenic granuloma* (pregnancy epulis). Such lesions are more likely to be observed in women with poor oral hygiene (as shown in Figure 20.3).

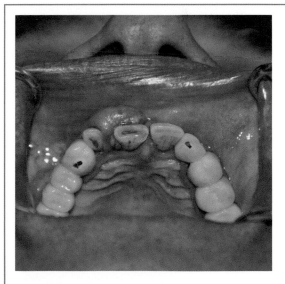

Figure 20.3 A pyogenic granuloma in the upper right anterior region in a 23-year-old pregnant lady. *Source:* Courtesy of Professor K. Ataullah.

Periodontal disease during pregnancy is associated with pre-term birth as well as low birthweight.

Genitourinary System

The actions of hCG already described on the cardiovascular system also have an effect on other organs, such as the kidneys. The rate of blood flow through the kidney governs the filtration rate, so if blood flow increases, the glomerular filtration rate does too – by up to 60–70% in pregnancy, leading to women complaining of polyuria from six weeks.

Dilatation of the ureter may result from compression from the enlarging uterus and hypotonia due to progesterone. This leads to urinary stasis which accounts for an increased risk of urinary tract infections during pregnancy.

Haematologic System

Pregnancy is associated with an up to 20% increase in red cell mass and a 25–50% increase in blood volume compared to non-pregnant women by late pregnancy. The disproportionate increase in blood volume results in haemodilution and physiologic anaemia reducing the haematocrit to less than 40% of the non-pregnant value.

Pregnancy is also associated with an increase in clotting factors and a decrease in fibrinolytic activity, producing a hypercoagulable state. Moreover, venous stasis may result from the compression of inferior vena cava and iliac veins by the gravid uterus. These aforementioned changes increase the risk of thromboembolism by up to fivefold. Pulmonary embolism from deep venous thrombosis has a high risk of sudden death.

Other Considerations

Maternal infections and nutritional deficiencies during pregnancy may lead to adverse effects on the developing dentition of the foetus, including enamel hypoplasia.

Elective dental treatment should be avoided during pregnancy, especially during the first trimester, owing to the potential risk of miscarriage. Furthermore, as it is a period of organogenesis, the developing embryo is particularly vulnerable to harmful effects of drugs. Thus, if dental treatment is required, it is best provided during the second trimester.

Drugs routinely prescribed during dental treatment should be re-evaluated during pregnancy and lactation for potential risks to the mother and foetus/newborn. Local anaesthetics may be administered during pregnancy, if indicated. However, the dose must be kept to a minimum and aspiration is mandatory to avoid intravascular injections and consequent systemic toxicity. Analgesics and antibiotics should also be used only when absolutely essential. Use of tetracycline antibiotics during pregnancy or lactation may lead to permanent staining of the teeth in the foetus/newborn.

Reference

Tortora, G.J. and Derrickson, B. (2013). *Principles of Anatomy and Physiology*. Hoboken, NJ: Wiley.

Further Reading

Hall, J.E. (2015). Chapters 82 and 83. In: *Guyton and Hall Textbook of Medical Physiology*, 13e. Philadelphia: Elsevier.

Hasudungan, A. (2018). Female reproductive system: Menstrual cycle, hormones and regulation. https://www.youtube.com/watch?v=2_owp8kNMus (accessed 1 May 2018).

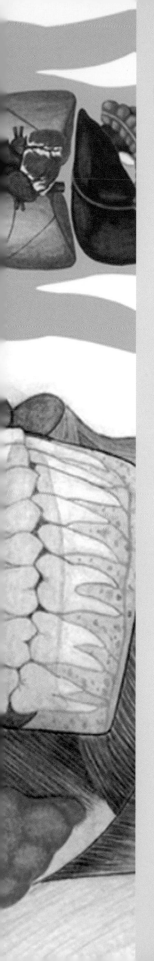

PART IX
Nervous System

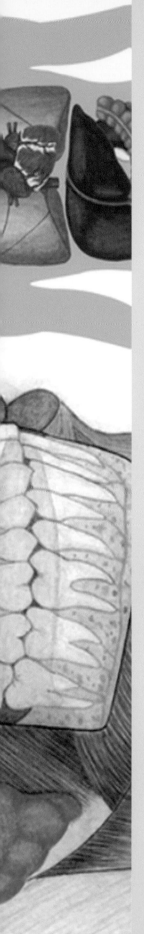

CHAPTER 21
Central Nervous System

Elizabeth Prabhakar and Kamran Ali

Introduction

The nervous system (NS) is a rapid communication system which controls the biological processes in the body. It serves as a processing centre for the integration of sensory, motor, and visceral function as well as higher-order functions such as emotion, thought, learning, memory, and intelligence.

The NS is composed of two main types of cells: *neurons* and *neuroglia*. Neurons are excitable cells involved in the reception and conduction of nerve signals (Chapter 2). The second type are the non-excitable supporting cells collectively known as *neuroglial cells*. The latter include: *astrocytes*, which are star-shaped cells involved in the transport of neurotransmitters; *oligodendrocytes*, which produce the myelin sheath for neurons in the brain and spinal cord (the myelin sheath for peripheral neurons is provided by Schwann cells); *microglia*, which have a phagocytic function; and *ependymal* cells, which line the ventricles of the brain.

The functional unit of the NS is the *neural network* (composed of individual neurons), because even the most basic functions require a circuit of neurons. An estimated 86–100 billion neurons link together to form extensive and intricate networks, which converge and diverge into producing myriad possible signalling pathways.

Divisions of the Nervous System

The NS can be divided into the central nervous system (CNS) and the peripheral nervous system (PNS). The CNS comprises the brain and spinal cord and the PNS comprises all nervous tissue lying outside the CNS. These include the cranial and spinal nerves, emanating from the spinal cord, autonomic ganglia, enteric plexuses, and sensory receptors in the skin (Figure 21.1).

Essential Physiology for Dental Students, First Edition. Edited by Kamran Ali and Elizabeth Prabhakar.
© 2019 John Wiley & Sons Ltd. Published 2019 by John Wiley & Sons Ltd.
Companion website: www.wiley.com/go/ali/physiology

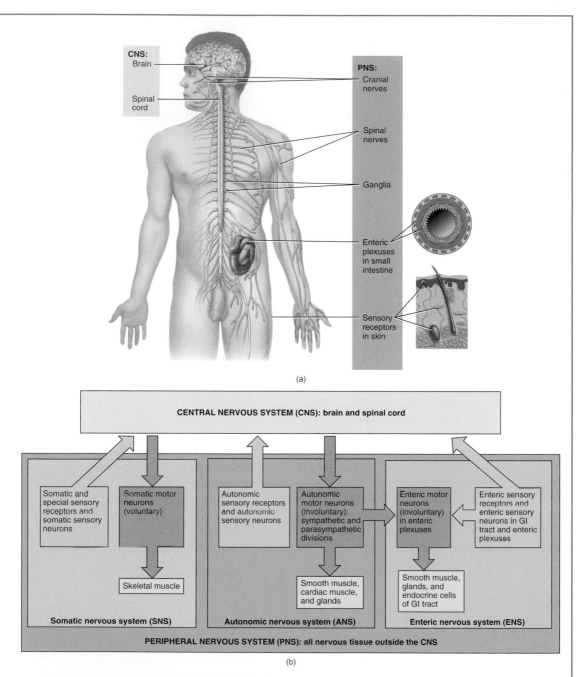

(a)

(b)

Figure 21.1 (a) Major divisions of the nervous system: central nervous system, CNS (beige) and peripheral nervous system, PNS (purple). (b) The CNS is divided into the brain and spinal cord. The PNS is subdivided into the afferent or sensory and efferent or motor divisions. The afferent division (blue) conveys information from the periphery via somatic, autonomic, and enteric neurons and receptors, sensory and visceral stimuli. The efferent division (brown) sends information from the CNS to the periphery, via somatic, autonomic, and enteric divisions to the effector organs, like muscles and glands. *Source:* Tortora and Derrickson (2017).

The NS is categorised into two pathways: the (i) afferent (sensory) pathway, sending sensory input to the brain and spinal cord, from the neurons and receptors of the somatic, special sensory, autonomic, and enteric systems, and (ii) the efferent (motor) pathway, sending output from the brain and spinal cord to the peripheral regions of the body. The efferent division is further divided into the somatic (SNS) and autonomic (ANS) nervous systems, which supply the effector organs or motor units of the body. The SNS is under voluntary control and innervates the skeletal muscle (Chapter 3). The ANS is involuntary is further subdivided into the (i) sympathetic and (ii) parasympathetic nervous systems (Chapter 22), which innervate the smooth muscles, cardiac muscle, and glands; and (iii) the enteric nervous system, which innervates the smooth muscles and glands of the gastrointestinal tract (GIT).

The Central Nervous System

The Brain

The brain consists of four main subdivisions: *cerebrum*, *diencephalon*, *cerebellum*, and *brainstem*. The cerebrum consists of the left and right cerebral hemispheres. The diencephalon consists of the thalamus, hypothalamus, and pineal gland (which encompasses the epithalamus). The brainstem, consists of the mid-brain, pons, and medulla oblongata, which elongates into the spinal cord (Figure 21.2). The cerebellum is attached to the dorsal aspect of the brainstem by three paired cerebellar peduncles (not seen in diagram).

Cerebrum (Telencephalon)

The bilateral cerebral hemispheres constitute a large proportion of the brain. A sagittal section through the

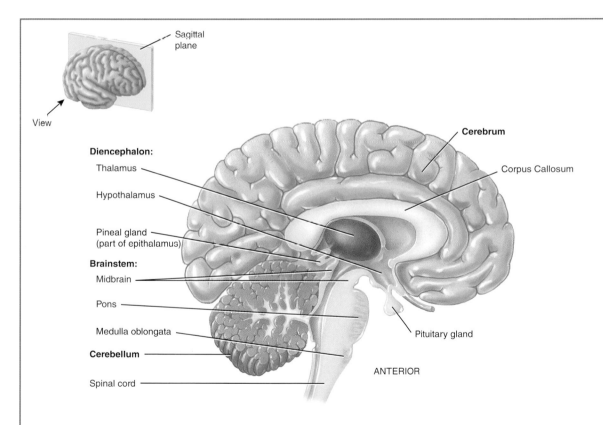

Figure 21.2 Overview of major brain components showing four major divisions: cerebrum, diencephalon, brainstem, and cerebellum. *Source:* Tortora and Derrickson (2017).

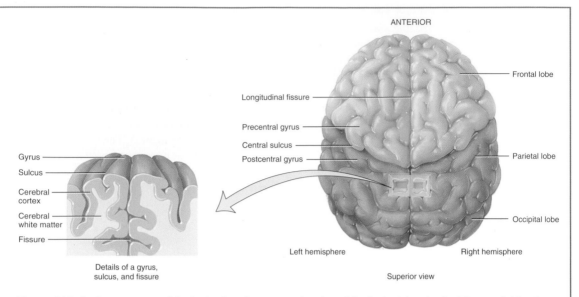

Figure 21.3 Surface anatomy of the brain. Anterior or superior view of the brain. A longitudinal fissure divides the brain into the left and right hemispheres. The inset shows that the surface of the brain is thrown into numerous folds or convolutions called gyri (singular gyrus) and sulci (singular sulcus). *Source:* Tortora and Derrickson (2017).

hemispheres shows that the cerebrum is organised into two distinct regions: the outer and inner layers. The outer layer is called the cerebral cortex, which is composed of grey matter containing the cell bodies of neurons. The inner region is composed of white matter, containing nerve fibres and neuroglia (Figure 21.3). The white matter of the cerebral cortex contains the *corpus callosum*, (seen in Figure 21.2) which connects the two cerebral hemispheres, and the *internal capsule* (contains ascending and descending axons to the cortex). The corpus callosum is a band of transverse nerve fibres (commissures or axons) which connect the cerebral cortex to the rest of the NS. Each cerebral hemisphere also contains a cavity known as the *lateral ventricle* (part of a network of ventricles in the brain) containing cerebrospinal fluid (CSF). The CSF plays an important role in protecting the brain from injury (acts as a shock absorber and prevents friction), providing an optimum medium for neuronal signalling (the slightest change in the extracellular ionic concentration would affect the generation of action potentials and postsynaptic potentials) and acting as a medium for the exchange of gases, nutrients, and waste products between blood and nervous tissue.

The cerebrum is divided into four lobes: *frontal, parietal, occipital,* and *temporal* lobes (Figure 21.4). These divisions are demarcated by the irregular external eminences called *gyri* (singular: gyrus) interspersed by furrows called *sulci* (singular: sulcus).

The central sulcus separates frontal and parietal lobes. The frontal lobe of the cerebral cortex is separated from the temporal lobe by the lateral sulcus. Immediately anterior to the central sulcus is the *pre-central gyrus*, which is the *primary motor area*. The *post-central gyrus* is located posterior to the central sulcus and represents the *primary sensory area*. The motor speech area is located in the frontal lobe above the lateral sulcus. The *temporal lobe* is concerned with auditory perception, learning, and memory, while the *occipital lobe* is related to vision. The taste area is in the post-central gyrus and extends to the *insula*, a buried part of the cortex adjacent to the deep aspect of the lateral sulcus. Each cerebral hemisphere is concerned with the sensory and motor functions of the contralateral side of the body, owing to decussation (axons crossing over to the opposite side; Figure 21.5).

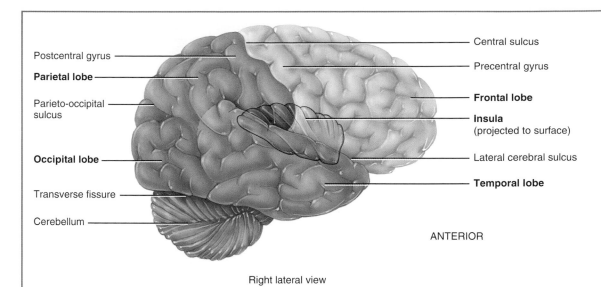

Figure 21.4 The four lobes of the cerebrum: frontal lobe, temporal lobe, parietal lobe and occipital lobe. The 'insula' is an area of the brain involved in taste sensation, which lies deep inside the brain. It is not visible externally and has therefore been projected to the surface of the brain. *Source:* Tortora and Derrickson (2017).

Primary Sensory Cortex   The conscious perception of sensation lies within the *parietal, temporal, occipital,* and *insular* regions of the cerebrum. Neurons within this area receive afferent information from somatic sensory receptors of the skin and proprioceptors in skeletal muscles (Figure 21.5, steps 1–5). The neurons are thus able to spatially discriminate or identify the specific body region being stimulated. The two cerebral hemispheres receive sensory input from the contralateral side of the body. As shown in Figure 21.5, sensory information from the right hand projects to the left cerebral cortex.

Primary Motor Cortex   The motor cortex contains large *pyramidal neurons* which control the precise or skilled voluntary movement of the skeletal muscles involved in handwriting (Figure 21.5, steps 6–8) or in manipulating dental instruments. The long axons, from the pyramidal neurons, descend to the spinal cord as thick motor tracts called *pyramidal* or *corticospinal tracts*. All other descending motor tracts arise from the brainstem nuclei. The pyramidal tract also receives 15% of its innervation from the premotor cortex (anterior to the precentral gyrus in the frontal lobe), which controls learnt repetitive motor skills. Any localised damage to the primary motor cortex (e.g. stroke) will paralyse contralateral body muscles, resulting in the loss of voluntary muscle movement. However, reflexive muscle contractions can still occur.

Diencephalon   Located below corpus callosum, telencephalon, and above midbrain, the diencephalon has a central cavity known as the *third ventricle* and has the following subdivisions:

• *Epi-thalamus:* Control of diurnal rhythms; links olfactory system to cerebrum (not shown in Figure 21.2).
• *Thalamus:* It is the largest portion of diencephalon and acts as a relay station for the somatosensory and some parts of the motor system (Figure 21.2).
• *Subthalamus:* Relay for sensory system (somatomotor zone of diencephalon), not shown in Figure 21.2.
• *Hypothalamus:* Integrating centre for the autonomic NS and endocrine system; participation in the visual system, Figure 21.2.

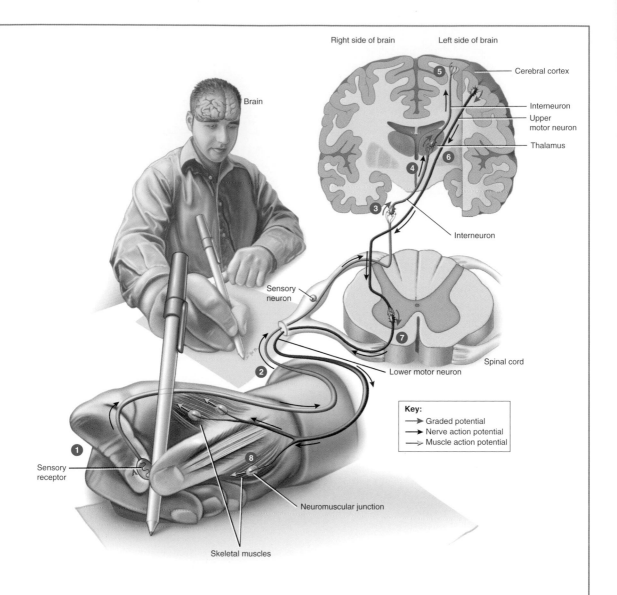

Right side of brain   Left side of brain

Cerebral cortex

Brain

Interneuron

Upper
motor neuron

Thalamus

Interneuron

Sensory
neuron

Spinal cord

Lower motor neuron

Key:
→ Graded potential
→ Nerve action potential
→ Muscle action potential

Sensory
receptor

Neuromuscular junction

Skeletal muscles

Figure 21.5 The afferent sensory pathway from mechanoreceptors in the right hand (used for writing or handling dental surgical tools) to the primary sensory cortex in the left brain (steps 1–5). The efferent pathway from primary motor cortex in left brain to the skeletal muscle in the right hand on contralateral side (steps 6–8). *Source:* Tortora and Derrickson (2017).

Brainstem (Rhombencephalon) The brainstem consists of three distinct regions: midbrain, pons, and medulla oblongata, containing the nuclei of the ten 'true' cranial nerves (CN III–XII). The expanded central canal in the upper pons and medulla is known as the *fourth ventricle*. The midbrain (mesencephalon) connects the cerebrum to the pons. The nuclei of the oculomotor and trochlear nerves as well as the mesencephalic nucleus of the trigeminal nerves are in the midbrain. The pons is located at the junction of the midbrain and medulla oblongata and connects the two halves of the cerebellum. Several cranial nerve nuclei are located in the pons, including the trigeminal (chief sensory and motor), abducens, and facial (motor) nuclei. The medulla oblongata is continuous with the spinal cord and contains the nuclei of trigeminal (spinal nucleus), vestibulocochlear, glossopharyngeal, vagus, and cranial part of the accessory nerves (Figure 21.6).

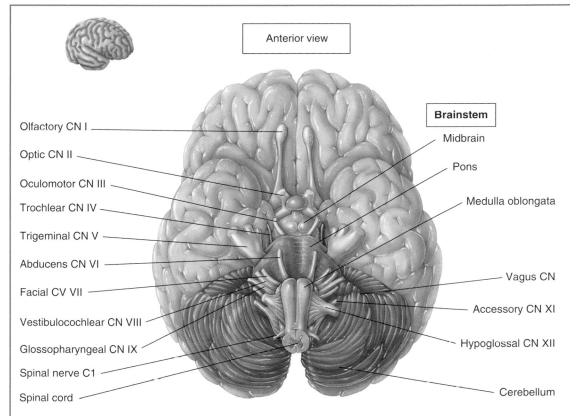

Olfactory CN I

Optic CN II

Oculomotor CN III

Trochlear CN IV

Trigeminal CN V

Abducens CN VI

Facial CV VII

Vestibulocochlear CN VIII

Glossopharyngeal CN IX

Spinal nerve C1

Spinal cord

Anterior view

Brainstem

Midbrain

Pons

Medulla oblongata

Vagus CN

Accessory CN XI

Hypoglossal CN XII

Cerebellum

Figure 21.6 Inferior aspect of the brain showing 12 pairs of cranial nerves (CN) in yellow. *Source:* Adapted from Tortora and Derrickson (2017).

Cerebellum

The cerebellum is part of the motor system involved in the unconscious coordination and fine control of muscles. It has a finer network of gyri and sulci than the cerebrum. It has two cerebellar hemispheres and central region, called *vermis*. The cerebellum is connected to the brainstem by three peduncles through which afferent and efferent tracts pass. These neural pathways are responsible for the integration and control of fine movements, the processing of vestibulocochlear (CN VIII) and proprioceptive afferents, and the modulation of motor areas in other brain areas and the spinal cord.

Spinal Cord

The brainstem elongates into the spinal cord. The spinal cord is a cylindrical structure enclosed in the vertebral column extending from the base of the foramen magnum to the disc between the first and second lumbar vertebrae.

The internal structure of the spinal cord is characterised by a distinct arrangement of the grey matter and the white matter. This can be visualised in transverse sections of the spinal cord, where the grey matter is condensed in the form of an H-shaped mass. The dorsal and ventral horns project from the grey matter bilaterally, marking the original of the spinal nerves. In the thoracic and sacral regions, a lateral horn projects from the grey matter bilaterally between the dorsal and ventral horns (Figure 21.7).

The *dorsal horn* is concerned with sensory function and contains several distinct regions:

• *Substantia gelatinosa* contains fibres mediating pain and temperature.
• Nucleus dorsalis (Clarke's column) relay proprioceptive impulses to the cerebellum.
• Nucleus proprius contains connector neurons (interneurons).

The *ventral horn* is concerned with motor function and contains the cell bodies of neurons

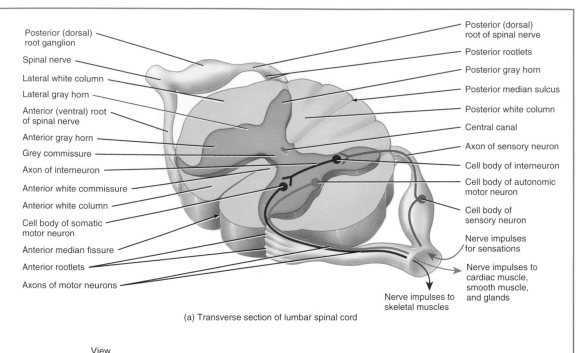

Posterior (dorsal) root ganglion

Spinal nerve

Lateral white column

Lateral gray horn

Anterior (ventral) root of spinal nerve

Anterior gray horn

Grey commissure

Axon of interneuron

Anterior white commissure

Anterior white column

Cell body of somatic motor neuron

Anterior median fissure

Anterior rootlets

Axons of motor neurons

Posterior (dorsal) root of spinal nerve

Posterior rootlets

Posterior gray horn

Posterior median sulcus

Posterior white column

Central canal

Axon of sensory neuron

Cell body of interneuron

Cell body of autonomic motor neuron

Cell body of sensory neuron

Nerve impulses for sensations

Nerve impulses to cardiac muscle, smooth muscle, and glands

Nerve impulses to skeletal muscles

(a) Transverse section of lumbar spinal cord

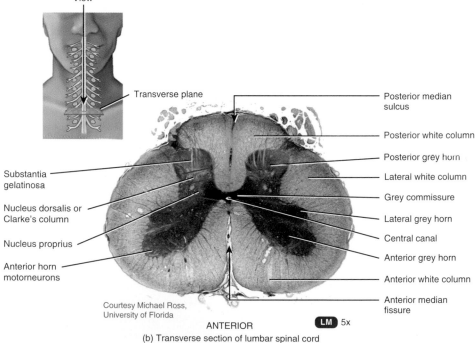

View

Transverse plane

Substantia gelatinosa

Nucleus dorsalis or Clarke's column

Nucleus proprius

Anterior horn motorneurons

Posterior median sulcus

Posterior white column

Posterior grey horn

Lateral white column

Grey commissure

Lateral grey horn

Central canal

Anterior grey horn

Anterior white column

Anterior median fissure

Courtesy Michael Ross, University of Florida

ANTERIOR

LM 5x

(b) Transverse section of lumbar spinal cord

Figure 21.7 Section through the spinal cord (a) showing white and grey columns (matter), the posterior (dorsal) and the anterior (ventral) horns, the dorsal root through which sensory nerves enter the spinal cord, and the ventral root through which the motor nerve exits the spinal cord (b) substantia gelatinosa, nucleus dorsalis (Clarke's column), and nucleus proprius. *Source:* Adapted from Tortora and Derrickson (2017).

which innervate the skeletal muscle (alpha motor neurons) and neuromuscular spindles (gamma lower motor neurons). The spinal nucleus of the accessory nerve (CN XI) is also located in the ventral horn of the upper cervical segments.

The *lateral* horn extends from the first thoracic to the second or third lumbar segments of the spinal cord and contains the cell bodies of the preganglionic sympathetic fibres to form the *thoraco-lumbar outflow*.

The second to fourth sacral segments of the spinal cord contain the preganglionic parasympathetic fibres, which together with the parasympathetic fibres of the cranial nerves constitute the *craniosacral outflow* (described in Chapter 22).

The Peripheral Nervous System

Cranial Nerves

Twelve pairs of cranial nerves (CN I–XII) arise from the brain inside the cranial cavity. Cranial nerves are numbered, anterior to posterior, in the order they arise from the brain. Cranial nerves are classified either as special sensory, motor, or mixed nerves (sensory and motor) (Figure 21.6).

Table 21.1 summarises the main functions of the cranial nerves along with basic testing in clinical settings. Cranial nerve testing must be done bilaterally when appropriate. The patient is initially asked for any subjective symptoms, which could indicate any sensory or motor deficit. This is followed by objective testing involving a methodical cranial nerve examination by the clinician.

Spinal Nerves

There are 31 pairs of spinal nerves (8 cervical, 12 thoracic, 5 lumbar, 5 sacral, and 1 coccygeal; Figure 21.8). Each spinal nerve is formed by the fusion of a dorsal (sensory) and a ventral (motor) root (Figure 21.7), and therefore are described as *mixed nerves*. The dorsal and ventral roots join before leaving the vertebral column through the intervertebral foramina. The dorsal root of each spinal nerve shows an enlargement (dorsal root ganglion) just before its union with the corresponding ventral root. The emergence of the spinal nerves supplying the limbs is marked by two prominent swellings. The cervical enlargement is related to the lower cervical and upper thoracic nerves and forms the *brachial plexus*, which supplies the upper limbs. The lumbar enlargement is related to the lumbar and sacral nerves and forms the *lumbar* and *sacral plexus*, which innervate the lower limbs.

Clinical Relevance

Facial nerve function may be impaired by several intracranial (e.g. stroke) and extracranial (e.g. viral infections, tumours, trauma, surgery) causes. Accidental administration of local anaesthesia during an inferior alveolar nerve injection may lead to temporary paralysis of the facial nerve. The upper part of the facial motor nucleus receives both crossed and uncrossed fibres; upper motor neuron (supra-nuclear) lesions lead to paralysis involving the contralateral lower third of the face. In contrast, lower motor (infra-nuclear) lesions result in paralysis of the entire face on the ipsilateral side.

As mentioned, facial paralysis can be one of the signs of cerebrovascular accident (stroke). Lives can be saved by learning to think and act F.A.S.T:

Face – has the face fallen on one side?
Arms – can they raise both arms and keep them there?
Speech – is the speech slurred?
Time – to call for emergency help (999 in the United Kingdom).

Other signs include:

- Sudden loss of vision or blurred vision in one or both eyes.
- Sudden weakness or numbness on one side of the body (including the leg).
- Sudden memory loss or confusion.
- Sudden dizziness, unsteadiness, or a sudden fall, especially with any of the other signs.

Damage to branches of the cranial nerves may result from trauma, surgical procedures, or tumours. Cheek bone fractures may result in numbness in the distribution of the infraorbital branch of the trigeminal nerve (CN V). Facial fractures involving the orbit may also lead to double vision (diplopia) due to paralysis of the extraocular muscles. The inferior alveolar and lingual branches of CN V are closely related to the lower third molar (M3). Surgical extractions of M3 may lead to temporary or permanent damage to these nerves.

Table 21.1 Distribution and clinical testing of cranial nerves.

Cranial Nerve Function	Testing
I OLFACTORY Special sensory to nasal mucosa (olfaction)	Check patency of nostrils bilaterally (sniff in) Expose each nostril to agents with typical odour (e.g. peppermint, coffee, lavender, lemon, soap) with the eyes closed and check recognition of familiar odours
II OPTIC Special sensory to eyeball (vision)	Best tested in specialist settings by an optician or an ophthalmologist Visual acuity tested using Snellen type charts Colour blindness tested using Ishihara plates Visual fields may be tested manually or by perimetry by an optometrist Ophthalmoscope may be used to check the optic disc, retina, retinal vessels, etc.
III OCULOMOTOR Motor (somatic) to the following muscles:	
Levator palpebrae superioris	Note any drooping of the upper eyelid (ptosis) when raising the eyeball
Superior rectus pulls eye upwards Inferior rectus pulls eye downwards Medial rectus pulls eye medially Inferior oblique pulls eye up and out	Note any asymmetry of the eyeball volume or pupillary levels Stabilise the head with left hand and ask the patient to follow the movements of your right index finger (in the form of H) sitting approximately 40 cm away at the same height Check eyeball movements and note any double vision, or pain during movements of the eyeballs
Autonomic to the pupillary muscles Dilatation (sympathetic) Constriction (parasympathetic)	Test using a torch 50 cm away Shine light in one eye and remove immediately; pupil should respond briskly by constriction and dilatation (II and III) Consensual response in the contra lateral pupil (less marked) Additionally, test using bright light in the room/dark room and note any difference between right and left pupil Finger movement toward the eyeball will also lead to convergence of the eyes and constriction of the pupil to prevent diverging light rays from hitting the periphery of the retina (accommodation-convergence reflex)
IV TROCHLEAR Motor (somatic): Superior oblique pulls eye down and out	As for oculomotor

Table 21.1 (Continued)	
Cranial Nerve Function	**Testing**
V TRIGEMINAL *Mixed Nerve*	
Sensory supply to face, scalp, and oral cavity including the dentition	Use light touch, two-point discrimination in the upper, middle, and lower third of face and oral cavity as appropriate Deep touch, pin prick stimulation usually unnecessary Corneal reflex (ophthalmic division of CN V) – usually not required
Motor (branchial) to muscles of mastication, mylohyoid, anterior belly of digastric, tensor tympani, and tensor veli palatini	Note muscle bulk on clenching teeth together (Masseter, temporalis) Check mouth opening and closure Jaw movements: protrusive, lateral Movements may also be checked against resistance
VI ABDUCENS Motor (somatic) supply to lateral rectus Pulls eye laterally	As for oculomotor
VII FACIAL Motor (branchial) to the muscles of facial expression	Lift the eyebrows to produce wrinkles on forehead; shut the eyes; grin, whistle, etc. Movements may also be checked against resistance
General sensory skin in external ear canal	
Special sensory anterior two-thirds of tongue:	
Autonomic (parasympathetic) to lacrimal, submandibular, and sublingual salivary glands	
VIII VESTIBULOCOCHLEAR Special sensory	Best tested in specialist settings: ENT/audiologist
Cochlear nerve (also auditory or acoustic nerve) carries auditory sensory information from the cochlea of the inner ear directly to the brain	Check hearing by whispering near each ear separately or Use a tuning fork; strike the tuning fork and hold it about 2 cm from the ear, asking the patient to tell you when it stops Place the vibrating fork on the mastoid process and ask if it is heard. If it is heard by bone but not air conduction, it indicates marked conductive loss. With profound nerve deafness, the patient may be hearing it by bone conduction in the other ear Weber's test (Marked hearing loss): Strike the tuning fork and place it on the centre of the forehead. Ask the patient in which ear it seems louder. The vibration is conducted through bone and it will be
Vestibular nerve carries spatial orientation information to the brain from the semi-circular canals	quieter in the affected ear

(Continued)

Table 21.1 (Continued)

Cranial Nerve Function	Testing
IX **GLOSSOPHARYNGEAL** Sensory and special sensory to posterior one-third of tongue; tonsillar region, upper pharynx and middle ear Autonomic (parasympathetic) to parotid gland Motor (branchial) to stylopharyngeus Motor to soft palate and pharyngeal muscles (pharyngeal plexus- IX, X, XI cranial part) Visceral sensory fibres from carotid body and sinus	Note the position of the uvula (central) Check movement of soft palate by asking the patient to say, 'Ah, Ah' Check if swallowing reflex Gag reflex – usually not required
X **VAGUS** Autonomic (parasympathetic) to mucous membrane of pharynx, larynx, thorax, and abdomen (up to second segment of transverse colon). Motor supply to muscles of pharynx – pharyngeal branch through pharyngeal plexus Motor to intrinsic muscles of larynx Sensory to mucous membrane of larynx: skin of EAM and external tympanic membrane Special sensory epiglottic region of posterior tongue Visceral afferent to thorax, abdomen, body, and arch of aorta	Note any hoarseness of voice Check movements of soft palate and swallowing as for CN IX Check cough reflex Hering–Breuer inflation reflex Vasovagal GIT reflex
XI **ACCESSORY** Spinal division is motor (branchial) to sternomastoid, trapezius	Note any wasting of muscles Sternomastoid: turn face right and left Trapezius: shrug shoulders Movements may also be checked against resistance
XII **HYPOGLOSSAL** Motor (somatic) to tongue muscles except palatoglossus	Note any asymmetry or wasting of tongue Check tongue movements: protrusive, lateral, superior, inferior Push tongue against buccal mucosa on each side Movements may also be checked against resistance

Physiology of Dental Pain

Pain is a vital function of the NS, warning the organism of potential or actual tissue damage. Pain is an unpleasant sensory and emotional experience influenced by psychological factors like past experiences, fear, and anxiety, for example dental procedures and beliefs about pain.

In this section, a brief discussion of pain receptors (nociceptors), conduction of pain impulses to the spinal cord via specific ascending and descending pain pathways, and the modulation of pain by specific chemicals are discussed. Lastly, we will focus on two types of pain: nociceptive and neuropathic pain (trigeminal neuralgia).

Nociceptive Pain

Central Ascending Pain Mechanisms and Transmission of Pain

Numerous pain receptors (nociceptors) are present in the oral mucosa, periodontal, and dental pulp. Nociceptors are sensory receptors which specifically detect noxious (harmful) stimuli (mechanical, thermal,

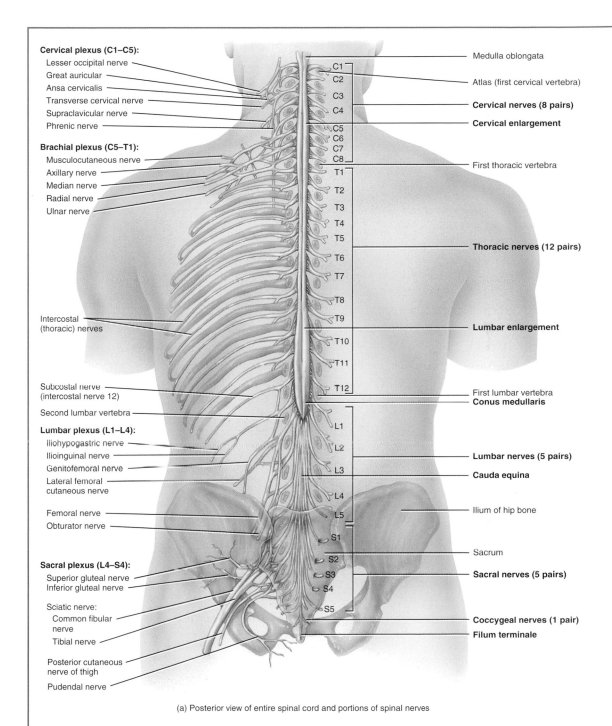

Cervical plexus (C1–C5):
- Lesser occipital nerve
- Great auricular
- Ansa cervicalis
- Transverse cervical nerve
- Supraclavicular nerve
- Phrenic nerve

Brachial plexus (C5–T1):
- Musculocutaneous nerve
- Axillary nerve
- Median nerve
- Radial nerve
- Ulnar nerve

Intercostal
(thoracic) nerves

Subcostal nerve
(intercostal nerve 12)

Second lumbar vertebra

Lumbar plexus (L1–L4):
- Iliohypogastric nerve
- Ilioinguinal nerve
- Genitofemoral nerve
- Lateral femoral cutaneous nerve
- Femoral nerve
- Obturator nerve

Sacral plexus (L4–S4):
- Superior gluteal nerve
- Inferior gluteal nerve
- Sciatic nerve:
  - Common fibular nerve
  - Tibial nerve
- Posterior cutaneous nerve of thigh
- Pudendal nerve

C1
C2
C3
C4
C5
C6
C7
C8
T1
T2
T3
T4
T5
T6
T7
T8
T9
T10
T11
T12
L1
L2
L3
L4
L5
S1
S2
S3
S4
S5

Medulla oblongata

Atlas (first cervical vertebra)

Cervical nerves (8 pairs)

Cervical enlargement

First thoracic vertebra

Thoracic nerves (12 pairs)

Lumbar enlargement

First lumbar vertebra
Conus medullaris

Lumbar nerves (5 pairs)

Cauda equina

Ilium of hip bone

Sacrum

Sacral nerves (5 pairs)

Coccygeal nerves (1 pair)
Filum terminale

(a) Posterior view of entire spinal cord and portions of spinal nerves

Figure 21.8 The spinal cord and spinal nerves. A total of 31 pairs of spinal nerves, originate from different levels of the spinal cord: 8 cervical, 12 thoracic, 5 lumbar, 5 sacral and 1 coccygeal. Spinal nerves are mixed nerves formed by the fusion of the dorsal (sensory) and a ventral (motor) roots. *Source:* Tortora and Derrickson (2017).

chemical). The pain receptors are free nerve endings, which transduce noxious stimuli into electrical signals or *action potentials* (Chapter 2) via the primary afferent Aδ and C-fibres to the CNS. The myelinated Aδ fibres are responsible for the initial reflex response to acute pain and transmit sharp, rapid pain. The small unmyelinated C-fibres are slow conducting and carry slow, burning pain. C-fibres are polymodal and are activated by chemical (e.g. capsaicin, found in chillies), mechanical, and thermal stimuli.

Damaged tissues also release inflammatory mediators, such as histamine, serotonin, cytokines, bradykinin, prostaglandins, substance P, or H^+, which can directly stimulate nociceptors or 'sensitise' surrounding tissues, by decreasing the 'activation threshold' at which action potentials are evoked.

Pain sensation is transmitted from the orofacial region by the main maxillary (CN-V_2) and mandibular (CN-V_3) branches of the trigeminal nerve, CN-V to the primary somatosensory cortex via a three-neuron relay, of first-order, second-order, and third-order neurons (Figure 21.9).

The cell bodies of the *first-order neurons* (nociceptors) are located in the trigeminal ganglion. Their Aδ and C-fibre axons leave the trigeminal ganglion and travel in parallel along with other facial sensory fibres (of CN-VII, IX, and X) via the spinal tract downwards to the spinal nuclei of the trigeminal nerve (located in the dorsal horn of spinal cord at the level of the medulla). In the medulla, the primary afferents synapse with *second-order neurons*. Both primary afferents, Aδ and C-fibres,

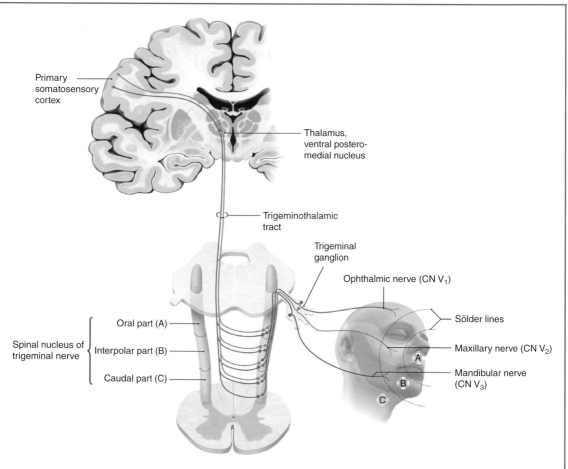

Figure 21.9 Pain pathways in the head and face. *Source:* Schuenke, Schultze, and Schumacher (2015).

branch to innervate nociceptive neurons in the *substantia gelatinosa* of the dorsal horn. The primary afferents also release a number of excitatory neurotransmitters including glutamate and substance P at their synapses with the second-order neurons in the thalamus (where transduction of chemical signals to electrical impulses occur, see synaptic transmission in Chapter 3), to transmit pain impulses.

Thus, primary afferents synapse with second-order neurons in the thalamus.

Axons of thalamic or second-order neurons (secondary afferents), collectively known as *nucleus proprius*, ascend to synapse with *third-order neurons* in the primary somatosensory cortex. There are two ascending pathways that carry nociceptive signals from the thalamus: (i) the *trigemino-thalamic tract*: the secondary afferents decussate to ascend to the contralateral thalamus, in the trigemino-thalamic tract, also called the *trigeminal lemniscus*; this tract carries the physical sensation of pain called *nociceptive pain*, and (ii) the *spinoreticular tract*: these fibres also decussate to ascend to the contralateral side to into the brainstem reticular formation (responsible for sleep, respiration, and alertness), before projecting to the thalamus and hypothalamus. This pathway is involved in the emotional aspects of pain which can make a person angry (by activating the emotional centre in a part of the brain called the *limbic system*), depressed, or unable to sleep due to the heightened alertness to pain.

Therapeutic interventions like nonsteroidal anti-inflammatory drugs, or NSAIDs, (e.g. aspirin and ibuprofen) or opioids (e.g. codeine and morphine) can be administered at different relay points in the ascending pathway to provide pain relief or analgesia.

Modulation of Nociceptive Pain In general, any pain is suppressed in the body via descending neural pathways, referred to as the *endogenous analgesic system* (Sessile 1987; Bingel and Tracey 2008). This appears to be a paradoxical situation since the primary purpose of pain is to prevent tissue injury or facilitate survival under normal circumstances. Modulation of pain can be explained on the basis of the two following theories "endogenous opioid mechanism" and "gate control mechanism".

Central Descending Pathway

Endogenous Opioid Mechanism The descending analgesic pathway is located in the grey matter of the dorsal horn of the midbrain called *periaqueductal grey matter* (PAG), which when stimulated produces analgesia (Figure 21.10). The PAG receives excitatory fibres from ascending secondary afferent fibres of the trigemino-thalamic tract. The axons of the PAG descend and synapse onto neurons of the rostral ventromedial medulla. Eventually, the afferents terminate onto inhibitory interneurons which synapse with second-order neurons (of the ascending pain pathway) in spinal nuclei of the trigeminal nerve.

It is thought that the central analgesic pathway modulates pain via the endogenous opioid system. To this end, the PAG and rostral ventromedial medulla contain an abundance of opiate receptors: *mu*, *delta*, and *kappa* subtypes (as do other central and peripheral nociceptive afferents), which bind to endogenous opioid peptides like β-endorphins, enkephalins, and dynorphins, to prevent pain transmission. Two putative exogenous opioids used routinely as analgesics in the clinic are morphine and heroin (the exogenous opioids are called *agonists* as they mimic the action of the endogenous opioids). The modulation of nociceptive input by opioids occurs in two ways: (i) blocking neurotransmitter (glutamate and substance P) release by inhibiting Ca^{2+} influx into the presynaptic terminal or (ii) opening potassium (K^+) channels, which hyperpolarise neurons to inhibit action potentials (Chapter 2).

There are functional differences in the distribution of opioid receptors within the CNS and PNS which may explain the unwanted side effects of opiate treatments. For example, the neurons in the respiratory centre of the brainstem have a plethora of mu-receptors, and inhibition of these neurons causes respiratory depression and may be potentially fatal due to an overdose. Opioid receptor action can be blocked by the drugs naloxone and naltrexone, which act as competitive antagonists (inhibitors) to opioid peptides.

Pain also stimulates the release of endorphins which block the ascending pain transmission to the thalamus and simultaneously activate the

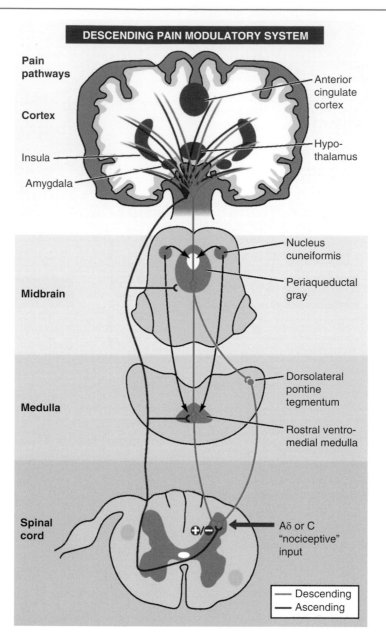

DESCENDING PAIN MODULATORY SYSTEM

Pain pathways

Cortex

Insula

Amygdala

Anterior cingulate cortex

Hypo-thalamus

Midbrain

Nucleus cuneiformis

Periaqueductal gray

Medulla

Dorsolateral pontine tegmentum

Rostral ventro-medial medulla

Spinal cord

Aδ or C "nociceptive" input

— Descending
— Ascending

Figure 21.10 Modulation of pain via the descending pathway (in green); +/− indicate nociceptive and inhibition of nociceptive responses at the spinal cord. Modulation occurs through the interaction between ascending (excitatory) pain pathway with the descending analgesic pathway at the level of midbrain, medulla and spinal cord. *Source:* Bingel and Tracey (2008). Available at: https://doi.org/10.1152/physiol.00024.2008 (accessed 1 May 2018).

descending pathways (Figure 21.10), according to Bingel and Tracey (2008), In addition, the release of a neurotransmitter serotonin (5-Hydroxytryptamine or 5-HT) in the thalamus and spinal trigeminal nuclei in medulla. 5-HT has the effect of modulat-ing incoming pain signals in the second-order nociceptive afferents, which synapse with inhibitory interneurons to block the release of excitatory gluta-mate and substance P involved in pain transmission. Thus, the systemic administration of opioids will cause pain suppression at the central and peripheral nociceptive sites containing the opioid receptors.

Gate Theory of Pain Modulation   First postulated by Melzack and Wall (1965), this theory regards *pain as a function of the balance between the information travelling into the spinal cord through large and small nerve fibres.* Pain can be modulated when there is simultaneous somatosensory input from non-noxious large Aβ fibres. If this input from the Aβ-fibres is greater than the noxious (nociceptive) input via the small Aδ and C-fibres, the 'gate' closes and pain transmission is inhibited. If, on the other hand, the noxious input via the small fibres is greater than those of the non-noxious Aβ fibres, the 'gate' opens to allow pain transmission.

The theory suggests that both large and small fibres synapse onto an inhibitory neuron in the dorsal horn of spinal cord, which acts as the 'gate'. In the absence of pain signals or if there is a greater stimulation of the large A-fibres, then the tonically active inhibitory neuron (keeps gate closed) suppresses pain transmission. If there is a strong noxious input, then the inhibitory neuron would stop firing tonically (to open gate) and pain would be relayed to the higher brain centres (Silverthorn 2017). Although the gate control theory cannot fully explain how pain is processed in the CNS, it has opened the door to new pain management strategies such as acupuncture and transcutaneous electrical nerve stimulation (TENS). Chipaila et al. (2014) have demonstrated that ultra-low-frequency TENS may be beneficial in the treatment of in non-odontogenic orofacial pain including temporomandibular joint dysfunction (TMD).

Clinical Relevance

Dentine sensitivity is common and usually results from exposure of the dentine due to tooth surface loss. *Pulpitis* (inflammation of the pulp) is characterised by severe pain and results from involvement of the tooth pulp by untreated caries or trauma. Painkillers only provide temporary and partial relief. The definitive treatment often requires operative interventions including devitalisation of the tooth by removing the pulp tissue (root canal therapy).

Trigeminal neuralgia may result from compression of the trigeminal nerve by tumours or anomalous vessels leading to severe pain as described in Chapter 2.

References

Bingel, U. and Tracey, I. (2008). Imaging: CNS modulation of pain in humans. *Physiology* 23 (6): 371–380. doi: 10.1152/physiol.00024.2008.

Chipaila, N. et al. (2014). The effects of ULF-TENS stimulation on gnathology: The state of the art. *Cranio: The Journal of Craniomandibular Practice* 32 (2): 118–130. doi: 10.1179/0886963413Z.00000000018.

Melzack, R. and Wall, P.D. (1965). Pain mechanisms: A new theory. *Science* 150 (3699): 971–979.

Schuenke, M., Schultze, E., and Schumacher, U. (2015). Sensory pathways: Pain pathways in the head and the central analgesic system. In: *Anatomy for Dental Medicine*, 2e (ed. E.W. Baker), 83. New York: Thieme Medical Publishers.

Sessle, B.J. (1987). The neurobiology of facial and dental pain: Present knowledge, future directions. *Journal of Dental Research* 66 (5): 962–981.

Silverthorn, D.U. (2017). Sensory physiology. In: *Human Physiology: An Integrated Approach*, 7e, 333–381. Pearson Education.

Tortora, G.J. and Derrickson, B. (2017a). The nervous system. In: *Principles of Anatomy and Physiology*, 15e, 404–440. Wiley.

Tortora, G.J. and Derrickson, B. (2017b). The brain and spinal nerves. In: *Principles of Anatomy and Physiology*, 15e, 477–525. Wiley.

Further Reading

Bozeman Science (2014). The Brain: Structure and function. https://www.youtube.com/watch?v=kMKc8nfPATI (accessed 1 May 2018).

Merritt, N. (2016). Pain control theories. https://www.youtube.com/watch?v=CQCQyHMu04s (accessed 1 May 2018).

Neuroscientifically Challenged (2015). 2-minute neuroscience: Pain and the anterolateral system. https://www.youtube.com/watch?v=gcOqv0uzyAQ (accessed 1 May 2018).

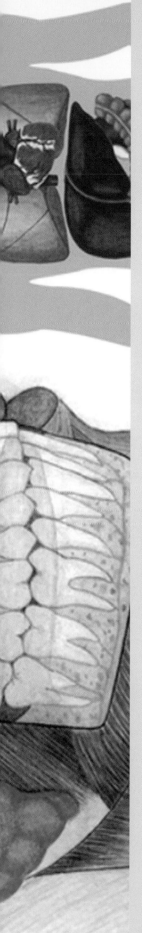

CHAPTER 22
The Autonomic Nervous System

Elizabeth Prabhakar and Kamran Ali

Introduction

The autonomic nervous system (ANS) forms the efferent (motor), automatic, or involuntary division of the peripheral nervous system (PNS). The ANS innervates smooth muscles of the viscera (organs), such as cardiac muscle, gastrointestinal tract (GIT), genitourinary system, glands, and adipose tissue. The autonomic innervation plays an essential role in maintaining homeostasis of the internal organs, e.g. baroreceptor and other cardiovascular reflexes, lung inflation reflex, and gastrointestinal reflexes (i.e. salivation, gag reflex). In addition to the normal homeostatic roles of the ANS, it also responds rapidly to stress, fight, fright, or severe pain, by coordinating simultaneous 'mass discharge' (initiated by the hypothalamus) of sympathetic impulses in all parts of the body, causing an individual to run away from unpleasant or dangerous situations.

Anatomic Organisation of the ANS

The ANS is divided into two parts:

1. the *sympathetic division*, which prepares the body for activity and is predominant during 'fight, flight' or 'stressful situations';
2. the *parasympathetic division*, which is responsible for specific or localised reactions and is active during the 'rest and digest' situation.

Most organs receive dual innervation from sympathetic and parasympathetic nerve fibres (Figures 22.1 and 22.2). The sympathetic fibres originate from the thoracolumbar region (T1–L3) of the spinal cord, and the parasympathetic fibres arise as craniosacral outflows (CN III, VII, IX, and X) and (S2–S4). The existence of the parasympathetic sacral outflow is currently being debated in the literature. For both sympathetic and parasympathetic nervous systems, preganglionic nerve fibres emerge from the central nervous system (CNS) to synapse within autonomic ganglia of the PNS. The autonomic

Essential Physiology for Dental Students, First Edition. Edited by Kamran Ali and Elizabeth Prabhakar.
© 2019 John Wiley & Sons Ltd. Published 2019 by John Wiley & Sons Ltd.
Companion website: www.wiley.com/go/ali/physiology

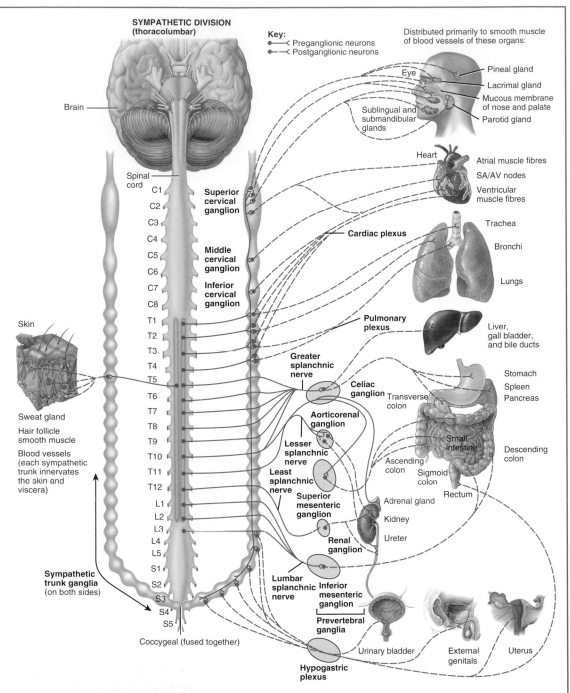

Figure 22.1 Structure of the sympathetic division of the autonomic nervous system. Solid lines represent preganglionic axons; dashed lines represent postganglionic axons. The preganglionic nerves exit from the thoracolumbar regions of the spinal cord to synapse with postganglionic fibres within autonomic ganglia. The ganglia on each side of the spinal cord, form chains, which run parallel to the cord (only left chain ganglia shown). *Source:* Tortora and Derrickson (2017).

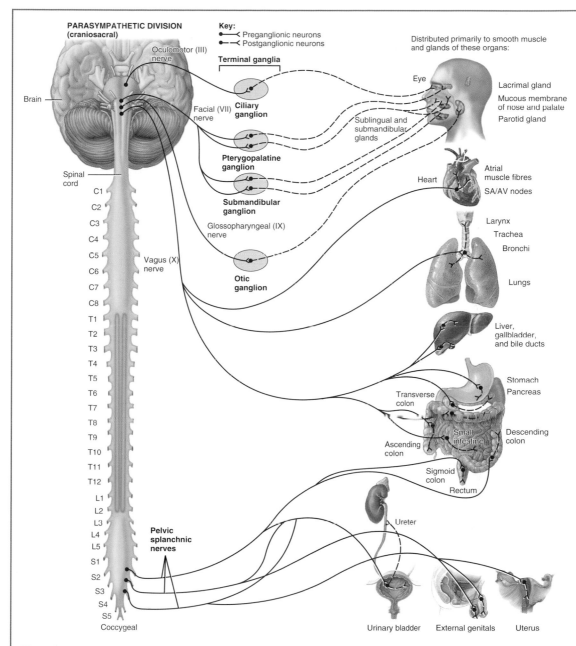

Figure 22.2 Structure of the parasympathetic division of the autonomic nervous system. Solid lines represent preganglionic axons; dashed lines represent postganglionic axons. The preganglionic fibres arise from the craniosacral regions of the spinal cord. The cranial preganglionic fibres enter discrete ganglia to synapse with the postganglionic fibres. The innervation of the organs is shown on one side only. Note the rich innervation of the orofacial region by the facial nerve (VII) and glossopharyngeal nerves (IX). *Source:* Tortora and Derrickson (2017).

ganglia of the thoracolumbar region form a sympathetic chain which runs alongside the spinal cord.

The arrangement of the cranial outflow of the parasympathetic autonomic ganglia is more discrete

(Figure 22.2). Once the preganglionic nerve fibres leave their respective autonomic ganglia, they are called *postganglionic fibres*, which synapse onto various target organs or neuroeffectors junctions.

Contraction, relaxation of relevant muscles or stimulation, and inhibition of glandular secretions in target organs are mediated by synaptic transmission (Chapter 3).

The preganglionic and postganglionic neurons of the sympathetic and parasympathetic nervous systems synthesise and release neurotransmitters; either noradrenaline (norepinephrine, or NE) or acetylcholine (ACh). Specifically, the preganglionic neurons of sympathetic and parasympathetic NS release ACh at their axon terminals. However, the neurotransmitters released by the postganglionic neurons of the sympathetic and parasympathetics are different. The postganglionic fibres of the sympathetics (sympathetic NS) release norepinephrine (noradrenaline), while those of the parasympathetics (parasympathetic NS) secrete ACh (Figure 22.3).

Therefore, based on the type of neurotransmitter released by the pre- and postganglionic neurons or the type of receptor(s) found in their target tissues, neurons can be classified as *adrenergic* or *cholinergic*. Adrenergic neurons release NE and cholinergic neurons release ACh. Similarly, those target organs which have receptors specific for NE are called *adrenoceptors* and those with receptors specific for ACh are categorised as *cholinoceptors*.

The adrenoceptors are stimulated by both noradrenaline (released from synaptic vesicles) and adrenaline released by the adrenal medulla into the bloodstream. Two main subtypes of adrenoceptors exist: *alpha* (α_1, α_2) and *beta* (β_1, β_2) *receptors*, which show varying degrees of responses to NE and epinephrine. The cholinoceptors also have two main subtypes of receptors, called either *muscarinic* or *nicotinic*. Both muscarinic and nicotinic receptor subtypes are stimulated by ACh. The receptors are the sites for drug action and are important during dental surgery (Figure 22.3).

The adrenal medulla supplements the actions of the sympathetic nervous system. The cells of the adrenal medulla are modified postganglionic neurons (Chromaffin cells), so called because they lack the fibres that would normally project to target tissues. Chromaffin cells are thus under direct neural control of preganglionic sympathetic fibres of the CNS (Figure 22.3). Chromaffin cells secrete neurohormones collectively known as *catecholamines,* which primarily consist of epinephrine, norepinephrine, and small amounts of dopamine. Upon sympathetic stimulation, catecholamines are released in the circulation and bind to adrenergic receptors of the viscera to initiate a widespread response (mass discharge).

Antagonistic Functions of the Sympathetic and Parasympathetic Efferents

The sympathetic stimulation is largely responsible for initiating the fight-or-flight response, whilst parasympathetic stimulation restores energy balance (rest and digest). Restorative actions occur through vasodilation of blood vessels supplying the gut, causing increased blood flow, motility, and gastric secretions. During digestion, the antagonistic actions of the sympathetic stimulation reduce blood flow (via vasoconstriction) in active skeletal muscles. Blood from the skeletal muscles is diverted into the gut. This autonomic control of GIT is regulated by the *enteric nervous system*. In the heart, sympathetic stimulation increases heart rate (positive chronotropic effect) and contraction force (positive inotropic effect). But, stimulation of the parasympathetics causes opposite effects (i.e. it reduces heart rate and reduces the force of the contraction). A summary of these functions and receptor types can be found in Table 22.1.

Sympathetic and Parasympathetic Tone

Both divisions of the ANS are continually active even without stimulation. This basal (normal) rate of activity in the ANS is called *sympathetic tone* or *parasympathetic tone*, respectively. The importance of tone is that it allows an increase or decrease in activity within a single nervous system (e.g. sympathetics). Sympathetic tone keeps systemic arterioles constricted to half their size. Stimulation of the sympathetic efferents beyond the basal rate causes further vasoconstriction. Decreasing stimulation of the sympathetic NS below normal causes vasodilation. Without sympathetic tone, only vasoconstriction but not vasodilation would be possible. This could lead to serious physiological consequences.

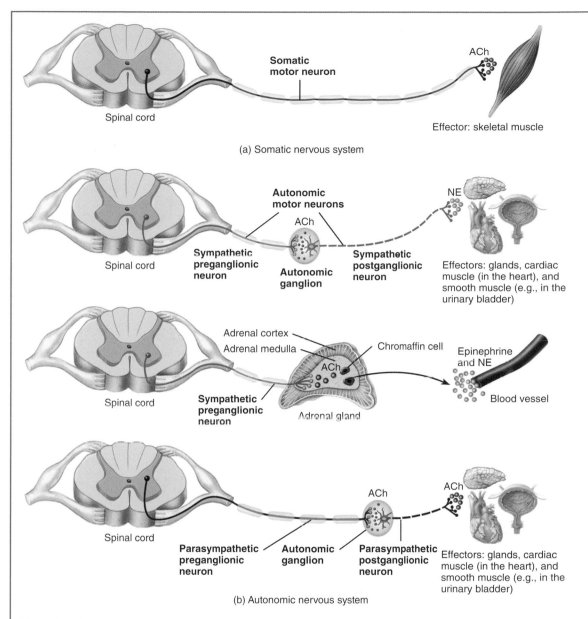

Figure 22.3 Neurotransmitter release in somatic (voluntary) and autonomic (involuntary) motor neurons. Preganglionic nerves (solid lines) and postganglionic nerve (dashed lines); (a) somatic motor neurons release acetylcholine (shown only for purposes of comparison with sympathetic and parasympathetic (autonomic) neurons; (b) sympathetic preganglionic nerve fibres release acetylcholine and postganglionic fibres release norepinephrine; parasympathetic pre- and postganglionic fibres release only acetylcholine. The cells of the adrenal medulla are modified postganglionic neurons (Chromaffin cells) because they lack axons that would normally project to target tissues. *Source:* Tortora and Derrickson (2017).

Table 22.1 Actions of autonomic nervous system.

| Effector Organ | Sympathetic (Adrenergic) Response | | Parasympathetic (Cholinergic) Response | |
	Response	Receptor	Response	Receptor
Adipose tissue	Lipolysis	β_1	—	—
Adrenal medulla	Increased secretion of epinephrine and norepinephrine, mediated via nicotinic ACh receptors	N	—	—
Alimentary canal and accessory organs				
Salivary glands	Vasoconstriction, increases secretions of viscous mucus and enzymes	α_1, β_1	Vasodilation, increases copious watery secretions	M
GIT				
Kidneys		α_2	Contraction – increased motility and secretion	M
Liver	Relaxation – decreased motility and secretion	β_1	—	—
Pancreas	Renin secretion	$\alpha_1 (\beta_2)$	—	—
	Increases gluconeogenesis and glycogenolysis	α_2	—	—
	Decreased secretion of insulin and digestive enzymes			
Blood vessels				
Arteries (most)	Vasoconstriction	$\alpha_1 (\alpha_2)$	No effect	—
Skeletal muscles	Vasodilation	β_2		—
Veins	Vasoconstriction	$\alpha_2 (\alpha_1)$		—
Eye				
Radial muscle (iris)	Contraction (mydriasis)	α_1	—	—
Circular muscle (iris)	—	—	Contraction (miosis)	M
Ciliary muscle	Relaxation	β_2	Contraction (accommodation)	M
Lacrimal glands (tear glands)	—	—	Increased secretion of tears	M
Heart				
Rate of contraction	Increase	β_1	Decrease	M
Force of contraction	Increase	β_1	Decrease	M
Nasal secretion	Decreases	$\alpha_1 (\alpha_2)$	Increases	M
Respiratory system				
Bronchial tree	Bronchodilation	β_2	Bronchoconstriction	M
Spleen				
Splenic capsule	Contraction	α_1	—	—
Skin				
Sweat (eccrine glands)	Increases sweating, mediated by muscarinic ACh receptors	M	—	—
Hair follicles, smooth muscles	Contraction (piloerection)	α_1	—	—

Table 22.1 (Continued)				
	Sympathetic (Adrenergic) Response		**Parasympathetic (Cholinergic) Response**	
Urinogenital system				
Detrusor	Relaxation	β_2	Contraction	M
Trigone and sphincter	Contraction – inhibition of	α_1	Relaxation – stimulates	M
Ureters	micturition		micturition	
Uterus	Contraction	α_1		—
Vas deferens/	Contraction	α_1	—	—
Genitalia	Contraction – ejaculation	α_1	? No effect	M
			Relaxation – erection	

Clinical Relevance

Vasovagal Fainting

Stress and anxiety associated with dental treatment (e.g. fear of dental injections) may lead to *vasovagal fainting* or *syncope*. Mediated by the ANS, syncope is the most common cause of sudden loss of consciousness, and up to 2% of patients faint before or during dental treatment. It is a biphasic response characterised initially by an increased sympathetic tone followed by activation of the parasympathetic system.

'Mass discharge' of impulses mediated by the hypothalamus stimulate the release of adrenaline from the adrenal glands into blood circulation, resulting in vasodilation in skeletal muscles (ß$_2$ receptors), leading to peripheral pooling of blood and reduced venous return. This is followed by vasoconstriction in the skin (α_1 receptors), leading to pallor and an ashen-grey appearance of the face; increased rate and force of heart contraction (ß$_1$ receptors). The vigorous contractions of 'empty' ventricles stimulate C-fibres in the left ventricles, increasing the vagal tone which overrides the sympathetic activity, causing a reduction in venous return and consequent cerebral ischemia. In the standing position, the *fainting* or *prostration reflex* helps to divert blood to the brain by causing the patient to fall to the ground: when the horizontal position is assumed, recovery soon occurs.

The vasovagal attack is transient and benign and rarely lasts for more than a few minutes. However, if a patient is maintained in an upright position in a dental chair, it could lead to permanent cerebral damage secondary to ischemia and loss of consciousness.

Therefore, if a patient experiences a vasovagal syncope in a dental chair, the chair should be reclined to make the patient supine and raise their legs to facilitate venous return. This simple manoeuvre helps restore the cerebral blood flow, allowing a rapid recovery within minutes owing to the antagonistic actions of the sympathetic and parasympathetic nervous systems via the baroreceptor reflexes.

Dental Local Anaesthesia

Vasoconstrictors, such as adrenaline, are frequently used in low concentrations in local anaesthetic injections in dentistry. The face and oral cavity have a rich blood supply and adrenaline helps to reduce bleeding during invasive procedures, increase the depth of anaesthesia, and localise the anaesthetics to the operative site, increasing their duration of action. Although adrenaline may cause an increase in heart rate, leading to palpitations, the effects are transient and usually insignificant. Conversely, inadequate pain control and bleeding during clinical procedures may cause stress and anxiety amongst patients, leading to excessive endogenous adrenaline secretion, which may far overweigh its dose given in local anaesthetics. Nevertheless, it is important to aspirate prior to giving a dental injection to avoid an intravascular injection accidentally. If adrenaline is injected into a blood vessel, it not only increases the risks of unwanted cardiovascular effects but may also lead to a failure to achieve adequate anaesthesia, owing to a rapid peripheral distribution of the drug. Finally, it is also important to limit the dose of local anaesthetics containing adrenaline to under 4 ml in patients with a history of cardiovascular disease or hypertension, and also during pregnancy.

Reference

Tortora, G.J. and Derrickson, B. (2017). The autonomic nervous system. In: *Principles of Anatomy and Physiology*, 5e. Wiley.

Further Reading

Costanzo, S.L. (2018). Autonomic system. In: *Physiology*, 6e, 47–68. Philadelphia: Elsevier-Saunders.

Guyton, A.C. and Hall, J.E. (2015). The autonomic nervous system and the adrenal glands. In: *Textbook of Medical Physiology*, 13e, 773–784. Philadelphia: Elsevier-Saunders.

Khan Academy (2018). Autonomic nervous system. https://www.youtube.com/watch?v=jA1NyCE4M2g (accessed 1 May 2018).

Pocock, G., Richards, D.C., and Richards, D.A. (2017). The autonomic system. In: *Human Physiology*, 5e, 182–192. Oxford: Oxford University Press.

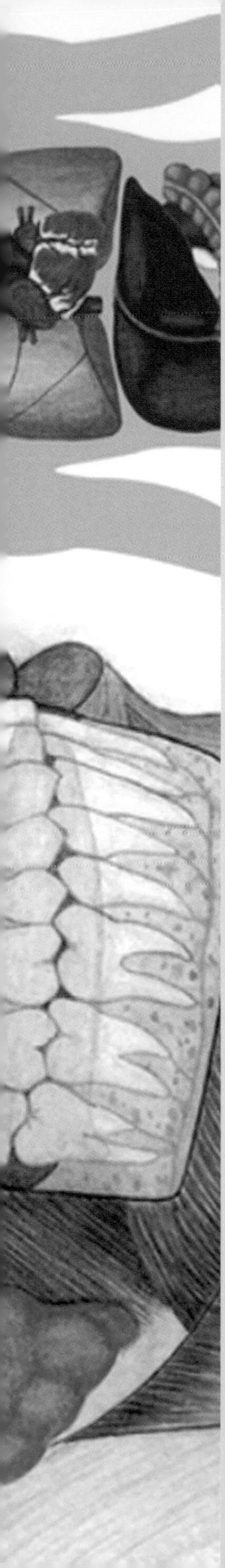

CHAPTER 23

Special Senses

Poorna Gunasekera and Kamran Ali

Key Topics

- Overview of the special senses including vision, hearing, equilibrium, smell, and taste.

Learning Objectives

To demonstrate an understanding of the:

- Structural and functional organisation of special sense organs
- Generation and propagation of nerve impulses in special sense organs
- Common disorders of taste

Introduction

Special senses are sensitive to stimuli that cannot be detected by the receptors of the general sensory system and thus have bespoke receptors that are specifically designed to respond to such stimuli. The impulses generated by special sensory organs are relayed to specific areas of the brain cortex that are distinct from the primary sensory cortex. The five special senses are: vision, hearing, balance (equilibrium), smell (olfaction), and taste (gustation).

Vision

The receptors for vision are paired spherical organs, the eyes, which can be described as fluid-filled hollow globes, and each one walled by three encircling layers of tissue (Figure 23.1). The outmost layer (fibrous tunic) is formed by the opaque white sclera, the anterior pole of which is continuous with the transparent cornea that allows light

Essential Physiology for Dental Students, First Edition. Edited by Kamran Ali and Elizabeth Prabhakar.
© 2019 John Wiley & Sons Ltd. Published 2019 by John Wiley & Sons Ltd.
Companion website: www.wiley.com/go/ali/physiology

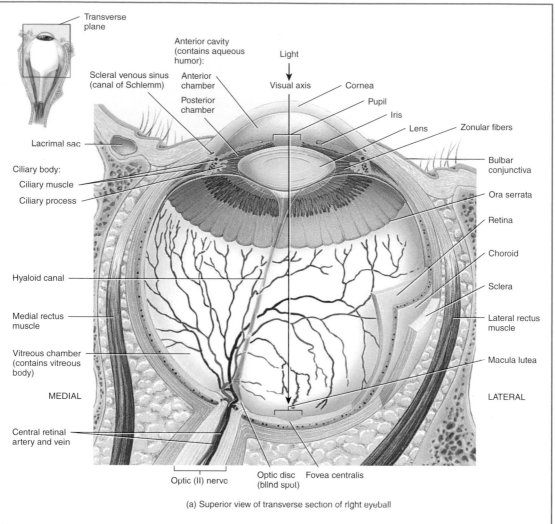

Figure 23.1 Anatomy of the eyeball. *Source:* Courtesy of Melina S.Y. Kam.

to enter. The middle layer (vascular tunic), the choroid, is densely packed with blood vessels and pigmented cells. The innermost layer (the retina) contains the photoreceptors that generate the visual impulse.

The iris, placed posterior to the cornea, functions as an adjustable filter for light. Deeper to the iris is the lens, which can change its curvature, facilitating an increase or reduction in the focal length. Immediately posterior to the lens is the vitreous humour, which mechanically stabilises the retina.

The light-sensitive cells of the eye, the photoreceptors, located in the outermost layer of the retina, consist of the peripherally placed rods (that respond to monochromatic light) and the centrally placed cones (that selectively respond to green, blue, or red hues of light).

Formation, Propagation, and Perception of Visual Impulses

Absorption of light waves by the specialised photopigments in rods and cones of the retina induces a change in the membrane potential of photoreceptors (Figure 23.2). This triggers action potentials within the optic nerve, which convey impulses towards the cerebral cortex. Only light waves that are between 400 and 700 nm in wavelength are absorbed, and thus referred to as the *visible spectrum of light*.

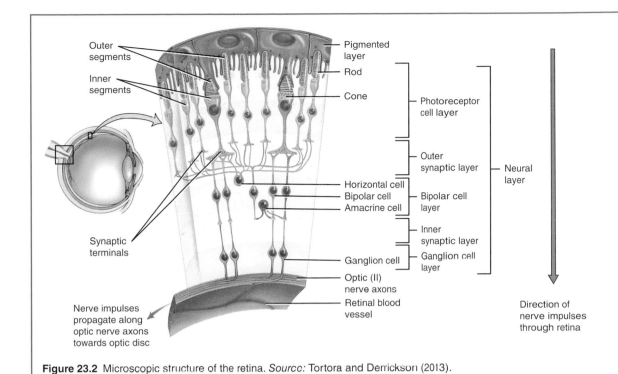

Figure 23.2 Microscopic structure of the retina. *Source:* Tortora and Derrickson (2013).

The optic disc, which marks the point of the exit of the optic nerve, also permits for the entry and exit of retinal blood vessels. The optic nerves exit through the optic canals and converge at the optic chiasm The neurons undergo a partial decussation to continue as the optic tracts to relay at the lateral geniculate nucleus of the thalamus. A final order of neurons from the lateral geniculate body relay the impulses to appropriate parts within the occipital lobe, which houses the primary visual cortex through tracts known as *optic radiations*.

Hearing

The process of hearing (auditory perception) relies on a specialised receptor: the ear. The human ear is made up of three linked compartments: the external, middle, and inner ears (Figure 23.3).

The external ear describes a funnel-like arrangement, responsible for capturing the vibrations of sound waves that are responsible for hearing.

The middle ear serves to amplify the intensity of these vibrations by up to 20 times. It does so through a set of three ossicles, named the *malleus*, *incus*, and *stapes*, respectively. One end of the malleus is attached to the tympanic membrane, which separates the external ear from the middle ear. The other end articulates with the incus, which in turn in attached to one end of the stapes. The other end of the stapes (the base) is attached to the boundary of the middle and inner ears.

An oval-shaped membrane (the oval window), to which the base of the stapes is attached, also marks one end of a coiled, fluid-filled, bony canal, located in the inner ear. This canal has a hairpin bend at its deepest point, with a second arm coming back towards the middle ear, to terminate in another membrane (the round window).

Both the round and the oval window are located within a few millimetres of each other, on the wall representing the boundary between the middle and inner ears. Both arms of this bony canal in the inner ear are filled with fluid, called *perilymph*. The arm of the canal connected to the oval window is known as the *scala vestibuli*. It extends to its deepest point, the *helicotrema*, from where it continues as the *scala tympani* to end in the round window. The outer surfaces of both the scala vestibule and the scala tympani are bony in structure, and are therefore collectively called the *bony labyrinth*. They

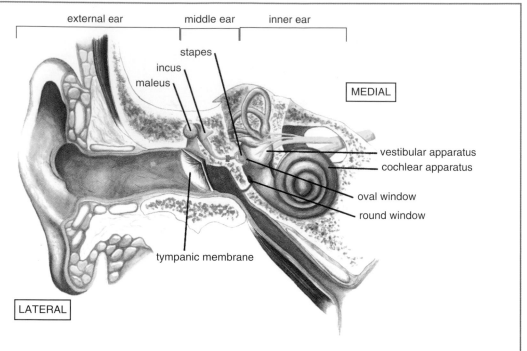

external ear middle ear inner ear

stapes
incus
maleus

MEDIAL

vestibular apparatus
cochlear apparatus

oval window
round window

tympanic membrane

LATERAL

Figure 23.3 Anatomy of the ear. *Source:* Courtesy of Melina S.Y. Kam.

are separated from each other on the inner surface by a blind-ended, fluid-filled (endolymph), membranous tube, the *scala media*, also known as the *cochlear duct*. The membrane separating the scala vestibuli and the scala media is known as the *vestibular membrane*; the *basilar membrane* separates the other surface of the scala media from the scala tympani. This arrangement of three canals, the outer two being continuous with each other at one end, sandwiching a blind-ended middle canal between them, undergoes a combined two-and-three-quarter twists preserving their relationship to one another. It forms the snail-like *cochlear apparatus*, which is responsible for the generation of auditory impulses.

The tissue which generates the auditory impulses, is known as the *organ of Corti*, which rests on the basilar membrane forming the floor of the cochlear duct (scala media). The organ of Corti is made up of about 15 000 hair cells, which are arranged along the length of the cochlear duct. While the base of each hair cell is firmly anchored to the basilar membrane, their apices are covered by about 100 actin-stiffened microvilli, known as *stereocilia*. The tips of these

stereocilia are connected to one another by cell adhesion molecules called *tip links*. This arrangement facilitates the stereocilia to sway in unison, very much like seaweed in response to water currents.

Formation, Propagation, and Perception of Auditory Impulses

The amplified vibrations transmitted to the perilymph through the oval window will travel along the scala vestibuli and continue through the helicotrema to the scala tympani to set off a corresponding movement in the membranous round window, if they are outside the frequencies that a human is capable of hearing. If, however, they fall within the human hearing range, they will take a shortcut from the scala vestibuli to pass through the cochlear tube, crossing the vestibular and basilar membranes, to reach the perilymph in the scala tympani. This process causes the basilar membrane, and the organ of Corti attached to it, to vibrate in synchrony.

Overhanging the stereocilia of the hair cells in the organ of Corti is a stiff awning-like membrane, the *tectorial membrane*, which abuts into the middle of the cochlear tube. The stereocilia are pressed against this tectorial membrane, when the basilar membrane vibrates towards it, causing them to bend. This leads to an opening of the mechanically gated channels near the tips of stereocilia, to let potassium enter into the cells to initiate the neural process, generating an action potential. This action potential ultimately terminates in the primary auditory cortex, passing through a series of synapses, most notably in the brainstem and the medial geniculate body of the thalamus. The nerve carrying the impulses is known as the *cochlear nerve*, which forms one part of the *vestibulocochlear nerve* (VIII CN). Though a human ear is theoretically capable of detecting sound waves within the frequency range of 20–20 000 cycles per second, they are most sensitive to those between 1000 and 4000 cycles per second.

Equilibrium (Balance)

The sensations of balance and the position of the human body in relation to gravity are also detected by a specialised organ found in the inner ear. It too generates impulses using mechanically gated channels, which are then carried by the vestibular component of the *vestibulocochlear nerve*. However, the central projections of this nerve are destined to mostly end up in the cerebellum, rather than the brain cortex. The specialised organ that facilitates this process is known as the *vestibular apparatus*.

The vestibular apparatus too has an external bony labyrinth encircling a middle membranous labyrinth (Figure 23.4). The main sensory receptors (the hair cells) are embedded on a ridge on one surface of the membranous labyrinth, and respond to mechanical bending by opening gated channels, which leads to depolarisation. However, there is no tectorial membrane to initiate the bending of the 20–50 stereocilia found on the apical side of each hair cell. Instead, the stereocilia are embedded in a gel-like cupula on their unattached surface. The inertia between the watery endolymph bathing the hair cells and the gel-like cupula in which the stereocilia are embedded provides the force required to bend the stereocilia to initiate the neural process, leading to a perception of balance.

The vestibular apparatus provides vital information for equilibrium and facilitates the coordination of head movements with those of the eyes and posture. It does so through a structural organisation

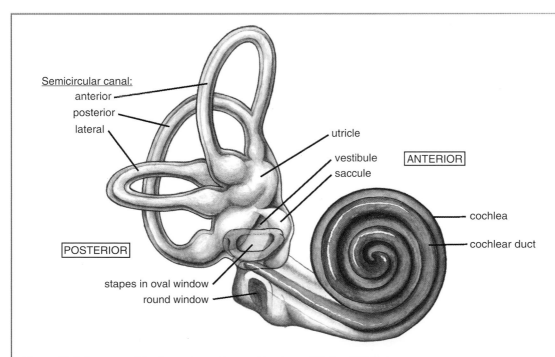

Figure 23.4 Structure of the internal ear. *Source:* Courtesy of Melina S.Y. Kam.

resembling a set of three semi-circular canals on each inner ear, which are connected to the auditory cochlear apparatus by two saclike structures, the utricle and the saccule, collectively known as the *otolith organs*.

The three semi-circular canals are arranged at right angles to one another; the two sets of semi-circular canals on each side are arranged as mirror images of one another. This arrangement renders them collectively capable of detecting rotational or angular acceleration or deceleration of the head in any plane, such as would occur with a sudden turning of the head, starting or stopping a spinning movement. The ridge-like ampulla bearing the hair cells are found at the base of each semi-circular canal.

The otolith organs, in comparison, are designed to provide information on the position of the head in relation to gravity (static head tilt) and rate of linear motion, as occurs when moving in a straight line, regardless of its direction. The gelatinous caps within with the stereocilia of the otolith organs are embedded are further re-enforced by minute calcium carbonate crystals (the otoliths), which serve to amplify the inertia between their movements and the surrounding endolymph.

The impulses arising from the vestibular apparatus are relayed to the vestibular nuclei in the brainstem and to the cerebellum, where they are integrated with those relayed from the visual system and proprioceptors associated with muscles and joints.

Olfaction

The olfactory receptor cells are located in the roof of the nasal cavity. The human nose overlies a central aperture in the frontal surface of the skull (the nasal cavity), which is placed between the two orbital cavities. It is made up of fibrocartilaginous walls, and divided into two halves by a flat central nasal septum. The walls are lined by a non-specialised mucous membrane, except at its roof, which is lined by specialised olfactory mucosa.

Olfactory Apparatus

The olfactory mucosa consists of the *olfactory* receptor cells and *supporting cells*, which secrete mucous that is vital for dissolving the odorants (molecules capable of inducing the sensation of smell) to be detected. The olfactory receptor cells have a bulging

cell body facing the nasal surface, from which a tassel-like arrangement of elongated cilia extends towards the nasal cavity (Figure 23.5). These cilia contain binding sites for odorants. The cell body also sends an elongated axon through the perforated cribriform plate of the ethmoid bone to the overlying floor of the anterior cranial floor, where it synapses within ball-like glomeruli found in the olfactory bulbs.

Formation, Propagation, and Perception of Olfactory Impulses

The neural component of olfaction starts when odorants bind to specific receptor sites in the ciliary process of olfactory receptor cells. This process favours odorants that meet two criteria: (i) they must be sufficiently volatile to enter the nasal cavity with inspired air and (ii) they must be sufficiently water-soluble to be dissolved by the mucous secretions of the supporting cells. The binding of odorants leads to a G-protein-linked cyclic adenosine monophosphate (cAMP) dependent cascade within the olfactory receptor cells. It results in the opening of non-specific cation channels, which in turn cause a depolarisation of the membrane, and generation of an action potential. This is relayed through the cribriform plate to synapse within the glomeruli, from which second-order mitral cells propagate the impulses to one of two main destinations: they may either pass through a subcortical route towards the limbic system, found especially in the lower-medial aspects of the temporal lobe (primary olfactory cortex), or course through the thalamus to the cortex. While the limbic connection explains the close link between olfaction and behavioural adaptations such as those evident during mating, feeding, and direction orienting, the cortical connection subserves the vital functions of conscious perception and fine discrimination of smell.

Taste

Taste (gustation) is the ability to recognise liquid phase stimuli and serves to communicate information regarding the chemicals which comprise ingested food and medicines. The combined sensory experience of taste and smell, along with the input from the trigeminal general sensory fibres,

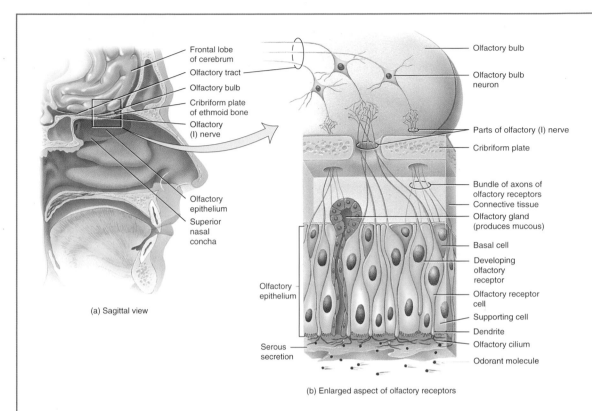

Figure 23.5 (a) Location of olfactory epithelium in nasal cavity. (b) Anatomy of olfactory receptor cells, consisting of first-order neurons whose axons extend through the cribriform plate and terminate in the olfactory bulb. *Source.* Tortora and Derrickson (2013).

determines the 'flavour' of ingested substances. Five basic taste sensations are recognised:

- *Salt* – such as ionised salts e.g. sodium chloride.
- *Sweet* – such as sugars, glycols, aldehydes, ketones, and some amino acids.
- *Sour* – such as citric acid, related to hydrogen ion concentration and degree of dissociation.
- *Bitter* – such as alkaloids (quinine, caffeine, nicotine), urea, and nitrogen.
- *Umami* (savoury) – such as glutamic acid and monosodium glutamate phosphate present in meat broth and fermented products.

The taste of ingested food along with the smell, texture, temperature, sight, and sounds of food preparation promote salivary secretion and prepare the gastrointestinal tract (GIT) for the digestion of food. Taste also serves to identify potentially harmful substances and, therefore, can also be considered to provide protection.

Taste Buds

Taste is a function of the taste buds, and in humans their number is usually between 2000 and 5000 but may be up to 10 000. Although taste buds are present in several locations, taste perception mainly involves the taste buds present on the upper (dorsal) surface of the tongue. The taste buds on the lingual dorsum are associated with mucosal projections, namely fungiform, foliate, and circumvallate papillae (Figure 23.6a and b). The filiform papillae, although most numerous, are lined by keratinised stratified squamous epithelium and do not contain taste buds. The filiform papillae perceive touch, temperature, and nociception and function as part of the masticatory mucosa. Taste receptors expressed in other locations throughout the body, including the palate, epiglottis, upper airways, and pharynx serve to protect the airway by initiating the cough reflex following an accidental entry of food. Moreover, bitter and sweet taste

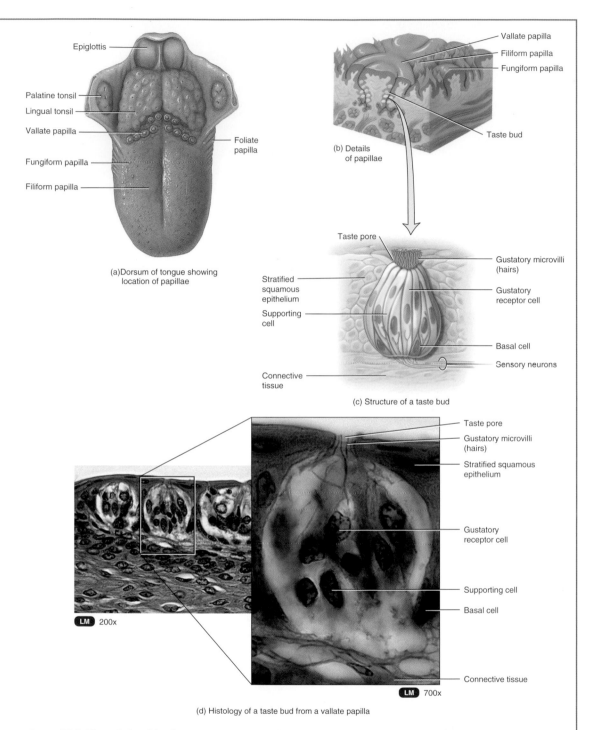

(a) Dorsum of tongue showing location of papillae

(b) Details of papillae

(c) Structure of a taste bud

LM 200x

LM 700x

(d) Histology of a taste bud from a vallate papilla

Figure 23.6 The relationship of gustatory receptor cells in taste buds to tongue papillae. *Source:* Tortora and Derrickson (2013).

receptors in the airway are capable of sensing bacteria and modulating innate immunity.

Each taste bud is an oval (barrel-shaped) structure embedded in the mucosa and is formed by a group of 50–100 neuroepithelial cells (Figure 23.6c and d). Each taste bud is separated from the underlying connective tissue by a basement membrane and terminates in a depression (taste pit) just beneath the surface of the mucosal epithelium. Microvilli from the gustatory cells project through a small opening (taste pore) in the taste pit and communicate with the exterior. Terminals of the gustatory afferent nerve endings enter the base and distribute amongst the cells of the taste buds for synaptic transmission.

Based on their morphology and protein expression, gustatory cells are categorised into three cell types:

- *Type I (Glial) Cells:* Characterised by an electron-dense cytoplasm and elongate, pleomorphic nuclei, these cells are believed to have glial-like functions and are thought to transduce salty taste.
- *Type II (Receptor) Cells:* Consist of electron-lucent cytoplasm and large ovoid nuclei, these cells express G-protein-coupled receptors (GPCRs) to mediate sweet, umami, and bitter tastes. These cells secrete adenosine triphosphate (ATP), which excites sensory afferent fibres and adjacent presynaptic taste cells.
- *Type III (Presynaptic) Cells:* Ultra-structurally, these cells are intermediate between type I and type II cells and possess synapses. They release serotonin, norepinephrine, and gamma-Aminobutyric acid (GABA). They primarily serve to transduce sour taste but also respond to sweet, bitter, and umami taste through cell-to-cell communications with the receptor cells.

Taste Mechanism

The taste stimuli are carried by the saliva to the apical part of taste cell membranes, which possess a variety of receptors, such as GPCRs and voltage-gated ion channels. Taste stimuli interact with the apical membranes of taste cells to alter the membrane potential. Once formed, the generator potential is conducted to the synapse and thence to the gustatory nerves (Figure 23.7).

Gustatory innervation to the anterior two-thirds of the tongue are derived from the *chorda tympani* branch of the facial (CN VII) nerve and distributed through the *lingual branch* of the mandibular nerve (CN V). Gustatory innervation to the posterior one-third of the tongue, as well as the circumvallate papillae, is derived from the lingual branch of the glossopharyngeal (CN IX). Finally, the *internal laryngeal* branch of the vagus (CN X) nerve carries the taste sensation from the base of the tongue and epiglottis.

Gustatory input from the cranial nerves is transmitted to the ipsilateral *nucleus tractus solitarius* (pl. solitarii; taste nucleus) in the medulla oblongata of the brainstem. The fibres relay in the pons before being projected to the thalamus (ventral posterior medial nucleus) and finally to the gustatory area in the cerebrum (parietal and anterior opercular insular cortex) to generate the taste sensation.

Clinical Relevance

Hypogeusia (partial loss of taste) and/or *dysgeusia* (distorted taste) may be associated with xerostomia, respiratory infections, medications, hormonal changes associated with menopause, and nutritional deficiencies (vitamin A, B, and zinc). *Ageusia* (complete loss of taste) is rare but may result from damage to the lingual nerve (CN V) following trauma and surgical interventions, such as removal of wisdom teeth. This may lead to temporary or permanent loss of general as well as gustatory sensation in one-half of the tongue on the affected side.

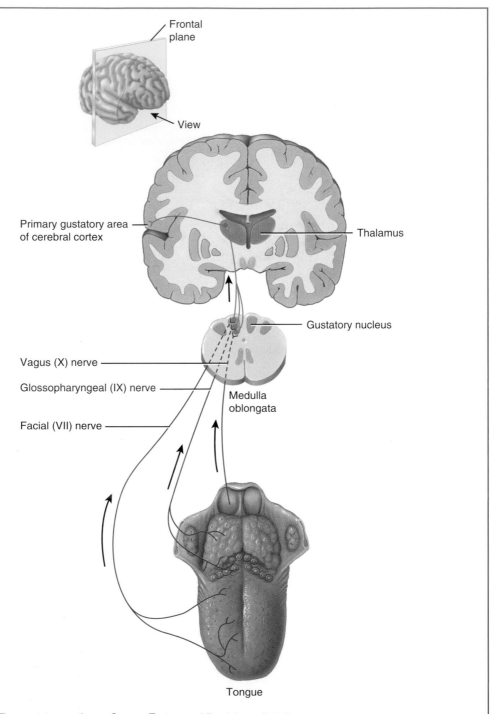

Figure 23.7 The gustatory pathway. *Source:* Tortora and Derrickson (2013).

Reference

Tortora, G.J. and Derrickson, B. (2013). *Principles of Anatomy and Physiology*. Hoboken, NJ: Wiley.

Further Reading

Ali, K. (2016). Oral mucosa. In: *Essential Clinical Oral Biology* (ed. S. Creanor). Wiley-Blackwell.

Dr Najeeb Lectures (2018). The human eye: Structure and functions. https://www.youtube.com/watch?v=fYwm4Ccj4Bs (accessed 1 May 2018).

Guyton, A. and Hall, J.E. (2016). The nervous system: The special senses. In: *Textbook of Medical Physiology*, 13e, 635–688. Philadelphia: Elsevier.

Khan Academy (2018a). Gustation: Structure and function. https://www.youtube.com/watch?v=-vp1X7_u3KU (accessed 1 May 2018).

Khan Academy (2018b). Olfaction: Structure and function. https://www.youtube.com/watch?v=5-McqAO8_Qw (accessed 1 May 2018).

Pocock, G., Richards, C.D., and Richards, D.A. (2018). The nervous system and special senses. In: *Human Physiology*, 5e, 218–267. Oxford: Oxford University Press.

SMC468 Graphic Design for Education (2015). Anatomy of the ear. https://www.youtube.com/watch?v=3G5jiXl2LSM (accessed 1 May 2018).

Tortora, G.J. and Derrickson, B. (2013). The special senses. In: *Principles of Anatomy and Physiology*, 576–621. Hoboken, NJ: Wiley.

Index

Note: Page references in *italics* refer to Figures; those in **bold** refer to Tables